The International Library of Sociology

THE DESEGREGATION OF THE MENTALLY ILL

Founded by KARL MANNHEIM

The International Library of Sociology

THE SOCIOLOGY OF MENTAL HEALTH
In 7 Volumes

I	The De-segregation of the Mentally Ill	*Hoenig and Hamilton*
II	Lunacy, Law and Conscience, 1744-1845	*Jones*
III	Mental Health and Social Policy, 1845-1959	*Jones*
IV	Mental Hospitals at Work	*Jones and Sidebotham*
V	Psychiatric Social Work in Great Britain (1939-1962)	*Timms*
VI	Put Away	*Morris*
VII	Social Service and Mental Health	*Ashdown and Brown*

THE DESEGREGATION OF THE MENTALLY ILL

by

J. HOENIG and

MARIAN W. HAMILTON

Routledge
Taylor & Francis Group
LONDON AND NEW YORK

First published in 1969 by
Routledge and Kegan Paul Ltd

Reprinted in 1998, 2000, 2002
by Routledge
2 Park Square, Milton Park,
Abingdon, Oxon, OX14 4RN

711 Third Avenue, New York, NY 10017

Routledge is an imprint of the Taylor & Francis Group

First issued in paperback 2013

British Library Cataloguing in Publication Data
A CIP catalogue record for this book
is available from the British Library

ISBN13: 978-0-415-17801-3 (hbk)

ISBN13: 978-0-415-86416-9 (pbk)

Contents

Acknowledgements

The research was carried out with the help of a grant from the Manchester Regional Hospital Board and we would like to thank Dr. H. Piggott, Chairman of the Mental Health Advisory Committee, and the other members of that Committee for their support. We further wish to thank Dr. J. S. B. MacKay, Assistant Senior Medical Officer, and Miss O. Allbeson, Administration Assistant to the Board, for their practical help on many occasions.

We would also like to acknowledge the contribution of Miss Nancy Young, Psychiatric Social Worker, who undertook the whole field-work of the project, and we are grateful to Miss Rose Glassberg for her help in preparing the bulk of the manuscript for publication.

Foreword

by

The Rt. Hon. The Lord Taylor of Harlow,
B.SC., M.D., F.R.C.P.

President and Vice Chancellor, Memorial University of Newfoundland, St. John's, Nfld., Canada

It is a pleasure to be asked to write a Foreword to this important book. Dr. Hoenig and Miss Hamilton have performed a useful and a valuable service in making a study of the work and effects of the psychiatric services in two typical areas in the Manchester Hospital Region. It so happens that, for fortuitous reasons, the Manchester Region has been able to pioneer in the new pattern of psychiatric care. For many years, the Region had been served by a few large and very isolated mental hospitals. Before the National Health Service came into operation, the people of certain of the county boroughs had decided that they wanted an alternative to this distant psychiatric care available at the time. As a result, comparatively small psychiatric units were established in a number of local authority hospitals. But they were no more than nuclei, with much of the old poor law atmosphere still persisting.

With the coming of the National Health Service, through the vision and foresight of Dr. F. N. Marshall, the senior administrative Medical Officer, and Dr. G. R. Pile, the Regional Advisor in Psychiatry, it became possible to upgrade and extend these units in a number of district hospitals to provide the beginnings of a model psychiatric service.

When the Ministry of Health introduced its ten-year plan, the development of the Manchester Region psychiatric units was already far advanced, and the whole of the Region is now covered by local units serving local population. Each is a comprehensive service for its area, making use of not only psychiatric beds but of full extramural psychiatric help. It is this complete integration of both domiciliary and institutional psychiatric services which is the aim of the present planning of psychiatric services in Britain.

Dr. Hoenig and Miss Hamilton have set themselves the task of assessing the effectiveness of this service and their results are both valuable in themselves and relevant to the needs of other Regions and, indeed, other countries.

Here is a pattern which, if successful, may have universal applications. It should result in a great reduction in chronic psychiatric care without an immense increase in the short-term services. I hope that the book will find readers wherever psychiatric services are being planned, and I believe it is one of the most serious contributions so far made to the study of this particular subject.

TAYLOR

CHAPTER I

Introduction

GENERAL

Comprehensive psychiatric units existing as departments in general hospitals are the final goal of a development which began around the time of the First World War (1914–18). By 'comprehensive' we mean a psychiatric unit which would deal with every type of psychiatric breakdown in a given catchment area and be in fact responsible for the care of any such case arising in that area. Since these units are located in general hospitals and have become part of them, they represent the complete integration of psychiatry into the caucus of health administration, the integration of psychiatry into general medicine.

Although there were voices raised and experiments conducted in this direction before the First World War, the major trend in those early years had nevertheless been towards segregation of the mentally ill. The administrative machinery, the medical services, the institutions themselves – all were kept apart from those connected with the physically sick, just as the patients themselves were. When the time came – namely, after the First World War – to reverse this trend, two aspects of the situation appeared as the main obstacles to change. One Jones (1960) has called 'legalism', and the other we might call 'bricks and mortar'.

The effects of 'legalism' have been well expounded by Jones (1960). She shows how the tendency to segregate psychiatric patients became incorporated in laws which gave these patients a separate status. Once part of the main body of law, they proved a formidable obstruction against any later attempt to narrow the gap between psychiatric and general patients or move towards an integration of psychiatric and general medicine. The statute which exerted the main segregative influence was the 1890 Lunacy Act. This brought into effect a Central Authority (which came to be known as the Board of Control [1913]), specially designated asylums to hold the patients, locked premises, and elaborate legal procedure governing admission and discharge. Many attempts were made after 1918 to bring about reform, but they amounted to hardly more than abortive attempts at modifying its influence. In fact, its segregative effect persisted and was really only overcome by the Mental Health Act, 1959, which repealed it outright.

The 'bricks and mortar' – the actual structures of the large mental hospitals, often so solidly built away from the dwelling-places of the community from which the patients came, and causing the removal of patients out into distant country – were the other expression of this segregative tendency, even more enduring than that of 'legalism'. The 'bricks and mortar' are still with us and cannot simply be abolished by the passing of a new Act of Parliament. To overcome this obstacle, other much slower measures will be required. Indeed just as attempts were made long before the Mental Health Act to modify the segregative effects of the Lunacy Act, so there were also attempts to break down the isolationist effects of the large institutions, and change their existing character. Efforts were made to alter them from custodial institutions into 'therapeutic communities' (Clark, 1960) and expand their activities through out-patient and day-patient centres into the communities they served. The most recent and probably the most radical attempts in this direction were enshrined in A Hospital Ten-year Plan for England and Wales (1963), which reflects the forecast made by the Minister of Health in 1961, that he expected 'the acute population of mental hospitals to drop by half in the next fifteen years and the long-stay population ultimately to dwindle to zero'. The Hospital Plan provided for a drastic reduction of psychiatric beds (by more than half) in the existing mental hospitals, and this would be only slightly offset by the proposed creation of new psychiatric beds in the general hospitals.

The Mental Health Act, 1959, seemed to have gone as far as was possible to counteract segregative tendencies by de-designating the traditional institutions and giving them the same status as other hospitals in the National Health Service. However, though the 'legalism' of the mental hospital situation could be dealt with in this way, the 'bricks and mortar' problem remained, a more enduring obstacle and a constant challenge.

The above development seen in historical perspective and in a critical light must not obscure certain positive aspects of the older régime. Both before 1918 and after, those who worked in the traditional 'lunacy' services made enormous contributions to the care of the mentally ill, all the more to be appreciated as they often had to work under difficult and adverse circumstances. Segregation itself was but a reflection of the climate of general opinion, the outcome of many fears and prejudices. That these were to some extent overcome was due mainly to the work of the most enlightened elements in this service, in particular the Board of Control, the statutory central authority, responsible for the patients under the Lunacy and Mental Treatment Acts. But individual doctors also and the educational activity of the constituent bodies of the present National Association for Mental Health have all made their contribution over the years to the growing sensitivity of public opinion to the need for radical change.

By the First World War the segregative tendencies of the lunacy legislation had led the psychiatric services into a cul-de-sac. The main disadvantages of the system came severely to light under the stressful circumstances of war, under which, according to Board of Control figures (1915), nearly half the medical staff joined the armed forces, which dismally depleted the mental hospitals. Nursing staff was also reduced and war-time privations brought the buildings into disrepair and affected the living conditions of the patients. It is interesting that it was conditions in a hospital in the Manchester area that, when these were brought to public notice, promoted the spark for administrative action. Jones (1960) describes these and subsequent developments very vividly. Dr. Lomax's book, *The Experience of an Asylum Doctor* (1921), which drew a grim picture of life in this hospital, caused such public agitation that the Minister of Health appointed a special committee to inquire into the administration of public mental hospitals. The committee made certain recommendations to improve the existing mental hospitals; it also created a public attitude more receptive to the earlier recommendations by the Board of Control for changes in hospitals in the direction of an integration of psychiatry with general medicine, and a de-segregation of the psychiatric patient. Indeed, the idea of treating psychiatric patients voluntarily in general hospitals had already been mooted at this very early stage. As early as 1918 the Board of Control had recommended both in- and out-patient centres in general hospitals for early diagnosis and treatment of psychiatric patients. At the time the public did not seem ready to accept this, but subsequent agitation over the Manchester hospital made society more receptive for administrative change.

The next important move came with the Royal Commission on Lunacy and Mental Disorder (1926), under the chairmanship of H. P. Macmillan. Here the stress was on the link between mental and physical illness as shown by various statements in their report, for example: 'it has become increasingly evident that there is no clear line of demarcation between mental and physical illness'. Further, mental illness was described as 'essentially a public health problem to be dealt with on modern public health lines'. No doubt these lines of thought were greatly stimulated by psychoanalytic thinking, which about thirty years after its inception had begun slowly to be familiar in this country. The Royal Commission wanted to see provision made so that patients could obtain psychiatric treatment without having to be certified; they tried to free a certain group of patients from the cumbersome legalism of the Lunacy Act, which they sought to have recast rather than repealed. At that time the Maudsley Hospital in London was still the only public hospital where in-patient psychiatric treatment could be given without preliminary certification.

In addition the Royal Commission were already focusing on other forms of 'de-segregation' for the psychiatric patient, mainly in the form of out-patient and observation facilities in general hospitals and of community care, by which they meant suitable social help for the patient in the period following his discharge from hospital.

As Jones (1960) notes, 'The Commission's recommendations as a whole marked a complete denial of the principles of 1890. . . . The legal view of mental illness was no longer acceptable, the medical view was fully endorsed.' The recommendations of the Commission were later incorporated in a somewhat attenuated form in the Mental Treatment Act of 1930. The main feature of this Act was to introduce voluntary and temporary admission to the existing mental hospitals without judicial order, thus making in-patient treatment available to a number of patients without having to submit them to the cumbersome and sometimes humiliating legal procedures. Even voluntary patients, however, were notifiable to the Board of Control, who still supervised these designated hospitals. The Mental Treatment Act, therefore, while attempting to reduce the segregative elements in psychiatric care only achieved a 'half-way' house status for the psychiatric patient as regards parity of status with the physically sick. Nevertheless, the ground was to some extent prepared by this Act for more rapid developments later on. These were again to take place as the results of war, the Second World War (1939–45).

During this war Dr. Aubrey Lewis (later Sir Aubrey) invited Dr. Carlos P. Blacker to survey the psychiatric resources of the country as a basis for future planning. The report was published in 1946 (Blacker, 1946). He recommended that there should be closer links between general and mental hospitals, and psychiatric services should extend from the mental hospitals into the community, mainly through out-patient activity, in a much more systematic and vigorous manner than before. There should be psychiatric beds outside mental hospitals 'for such early and remedial cases as do not go straight into an admission unit of a mental hospital'. He recommended 100 of such beds per million population (0·1 beds per 1,000). He seems, however, to have had in mind small psychiatric units on their own, rather than psychiatric units in general hospitals, which was in effect a slightly retrogressive step, as compared with that suggested by the Board of Control in 1918.

During the war, also, preparation began for the establishment of a National Health Service. In April, 1943, the Minister of Health stated in Parliament that this new scheme for the health service would not include the mental hospitals – a voice from the past, which, as it turned out, was overcome in the Ministry of Health's White Paper of 1944 ('A National Health Service'). A joint Memorandum (1945) of the Royal Medical Psychological Association, the British Medical Association (Psychological Medicine Section), and the Royal College of Physicians stressed that 'the argument for treating psychiatry in all essential respects like other branches of medicine' was 'strong and conclusive.... There is everything to be said for making the administrative structure of psychiatry exactly the same in principle and even in major detail as that of other branches of the health service.' As Jones (1960) points out, the advantages of full integration had become manifest to all. But it had to wait another fifteen years and the extensive investigation of yet another Royal Commission (1954–7) before this was given statutory expression in the Mental Health Act of 1959.

Meantime, the National Health Service Act duly found its way on to the Statute Book, and from 1948 onwards in anticipation of the major repeal of the lunacy legislation a number of further steps were taken to bypass the old segregative psychiatric services. Experiments were set in motion to bring the care of psychiatric patients into line with that of the physically ill, and integrate their treatment and care with the general medical and welfare services as a whole.

These experiments fell into two groups. The first group comprised those that further improved the existing mental hospitals, finally eradicating the old asylum remnants, creating firmer links with general hospital out-patient services and in some cases inviting other departments, such as ophthalmology, neuro-surgery, geriatrics, etc., to move into empty wards or villas within the mental hospital and so turn the mental hospital itself into a general hospital (Smith *et al.*, 1963). The second group form the concern of this present investigation. They consisted in comprehensive psychiatric services located in and operating from the general hospitals of which they had come to be an integral part.

PSYCHIATRY IN GENERAL HOSPITALS

The comprehensive psychiatric unit established in the general hospital, as we shall describe it here, is new of its type, but it is not the first time that psychiatric patients have been treated in general hospitals.

The Teaching Unit

Certain types of psychiatric units have existed in teaching hospitals for centuries. In this country Brook (1964) reminds us that Thomas Guy made special provision for twenty 'incurable lunatics' in his hospital in the early eighteenth century. Other hospitals made similar arrangements later, such as the Middlesex Hospital, and Guy's Hospital once again in 1861 with the York Clinic, after the original provision of twenty beds by the founder had faded out. In the course of time many of the teaching hospitals had psychiatric wards, although by no means all of them. The wards were usually small and the units were highly selective regarding the patients they admitted. The purpose was not so much a service to the population of the hospital's catchment area (although a limited service was rendered inevitably), but teaching and research. It was not until 1963 that there was a recommendation from the Royal College of Physicians (the Psychological Medicine Committee) that *all* teaching hospitals should have an in-patient unit of eighty psychiatric beds within their own confines (Brook, 1964). These new teaching units were to be seen in a different light. Their main function, being in a teaching hospital, was of course teaching and research, but teaching requirements were only deemed to be met if the units were large enough to take in the whole range of psychiatric disorder and render services to the catchment area, not just incidentally nor in a limited way, but in a realistic and fully effective manner. Thus the public-service function of psychiatric units in teaching hospitals was now no longer of an incidental nature, but had become a fundamental requirement for satisfactory teaching. The recommendations of the Royal College of Physicians in London have now become Ministerial policy.

Observation Units

Apart from these developments in the teaching hospitals, another important experiment was the psychiatric observation ward in the general hospital. The Mental Treatment Act, 1930, enabled this development, and a number of such wards were founded up and down the country. Although an important part of the care of psychiatric patients, the observation wards had only a circumscribed function and never aimed to provide a comprehensive treatment service. They dealt mainly with emergencies, and, as the name indicated, were primarily 'sorting-houses' for further disposal. As, however, physical methods of treatment improved, particularly after the Second World War, it was to a certain extent the experience gained in these observation wards which stimulated the idea that relatively small units in general hospitals could provide effective short-term treatment for a large number of psychiatric cases (Hoenig *et al.*, 1958).

Comprehensive General Hospital Units

Is then the present comprehensive psychiatric unit in the general hospital the child of these preceding developments? Undoubtedly the experience of such earlier methods of working was here to be absorbed into the new units, but the conception of their activity was radically different. Maclay (1958) has described what actually happened on the establishment of these units:

> . . . owing to circumstances which I need not detail here, there are some psychiatric units of one hundred to two hundred beds attached to general hospitals. Each has its own catchment area from which it admits all types of mental illness and provides appropriate treatment. Each is linked to a big mental hospital to which it was anticipated they would send a stream of patients. To our surprise they are sending only a very small number and seem to be able to deal with their case-load without getting silted up. We are inclined to think that this is because the units are small, so patients get individual attention; they [the patients] are in the centre of the community so that they do not lose touch with their friends; there are no vast grounds, so they go into town for their recreation and attend local cinemas and football matches instead of special hospital ones. It would appear in fact that one of the most important trends in psychiatry is a change from a demand for more beds in big isolated hospitals to a demand for more adequate treatment in more suitable surroundings. It is improbable that any further mental hospital beds of traditional mental hospital type will ever be required, and to me it is certain that the provision of more and more beds is not the way to overcome overcrowding.

This was not a private opinion, since the late Dr. W. S. Maclay was at that time a Senior Commissioner of the Board of Control of the Ministry of Health.

Thus it can be seen that not very long after the introduction of these psychiatric units into general hospitals, where they were seen as peripheral extensions of the mental hospital, they had come to be regarded as more or less independent units, expected (and indeed able) to deal with every type of case (with only certain limited exceptions) without recourse to any long-stay mental hospital admission. This development was seen as an *alternative* to the more conventional mental-hospital-based service and, as Maclay points out, a radically new development.

The answer to the above question as to whether the comprehensive psychiatric unit in general hospital was the child of the preceding experiments is therefore in the negative. The new units were not early-treatment units, but saw themselves as committed to look after *all* patients *throughout* their illness, and since many psychiatric illnesses are chronic conditions and the sheet-anchor of care in psychiatry is still 'management', it meant that these units were embarking on a policy of long-term care in regard to many of their patients. As they had only a small number of beds, the question immediately arose as to how they could be prevented from silting up with an accumulation of chronic patients. The viability of such units depended on avoidance of long-term hospitalization and their success in keeping the patients in the community as much as possible.

When Brook (1964) reviewed the whole situation, the existing scene was a varied one. He enumerated at least six different possibilities for psychiatric work in general hospitals, and it must be remembered that the comprehensive psychiatric unit in general hospitals as here described and investigated is only one of them.

THE SPECIAL ROLE OF THE MANCHESTER REGION

For some reason Manchester and its surrounding Region was destined to play a 'star' role in development from the beginning. Once more we go back to 1918, when the Board of Control recommended the official encouragement of out-patient clinics in general hospitals, which they considered 'inseparably connected with the improvement of methods of dealing with incipient insanity'. Among the places that first instituted such clinics was Manchester.

Also in Manchester, it will be remembered, the disadvantages of the segregative policy of the pre-First World War era came to a head in the inquiry following Dr. Lomax's book. As mentioned earlier, it was this book which caused public outcry and prepared the way for subsequent developments leading to the return of psychiatry to the medical fold.

Having been one of the last strongholds of the previous régime, the Manchester area moved into the vanguard of the new developments after the Second World War. Smith (1960) wrote a review of the psychiatric units established in general hospitals in the area administered by the Manchester Regional Hospital Board. He says:

> Ever since 1948 the medical administrative staff of the Manchester Regional Hospital Board have very definitely stressed the value of the concept of units for psychiatric patients attached to general hospitals . . . they felt that with the advent of the National Health Service there had been provided great opportunity to reorganize the mental health service in the Board's area.

He sums up his account of the regional psychiatric scheme by saying: 'It will thus be apparent that as far back as 1950 a planned and coherent policy of psychiatric units was being envisaged not in a few isolated cases, but as part of a planned, integrated, and far-reaching scheme to affect the whole area.'

Following a survey by the Regional Board in 1948–53, Dr. Marshall, the Senior Administrative Officer (Marshall *et al.*, 1953), could also write: 'it can be claimed with some justification that psychiatry has now come to be recognized in the Manchester Region as an essential general hospital service'.

At the present time, indeed, one can no longer speak of 'an experiment' in regard to these psychiatric units, though development still continues. In 1962 a total of 23,226 new psychiatric patients were recorded for the whole Region (in- and out-patients); the total number for the psychiatric units amounted to 17,664 patients, i.e. 76·3% of new patients in the Region were seen at or admitted to the general hospital psychiatric units, and only 23·7% (5,362 patients) were similarly dealt with by the older mental hospitals. (From all these figures mental subnormality has been excluded.) It will be seen therefore that three-quarters of all new psychiatric patients

Fig. 1

MANCHESTER REGIONAL HOSPITAL BOARD

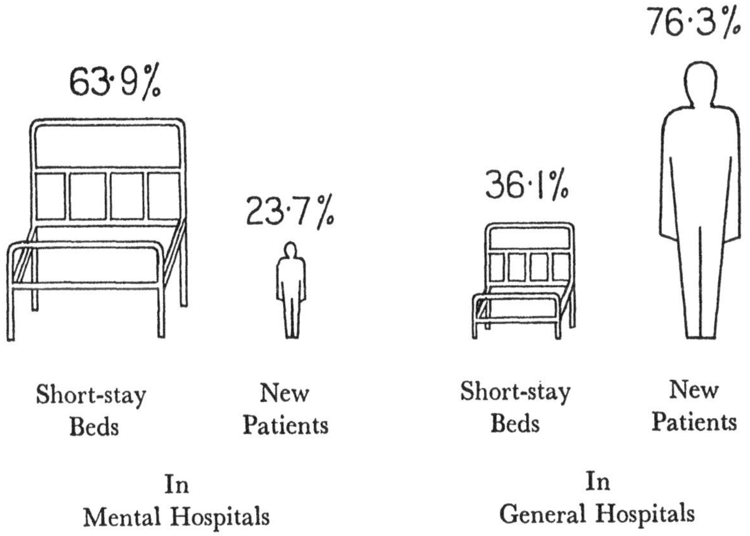

The figure shows the inverse proportion of short-stay beds to new patients between mental hospitals and general hospital psychiatric units in the Manchester Region in 1960.

were dealt with in the first instance by the new general hospital psychiatric units.

Nevertheless, if in-patient admissions are looked at separately, we find that mental hospitals were still playing a not inconsiderable part. The general hospital psychiatric units were receiving 6,374 new in-patients per annum (representing 57·4% of the regional total), while the mental hospitals were receiving 4,715 patients (representing 42·6%). Figure 1 illustrates how this relates to the existing number of beds. There were seventeen general hospital psychiatric units at that time with a total of 1,815 beds between them. This amounted to 15·5% of all the psychiatric beds in the Region. The mental hospitals had a total of 9,931 beds, which was 84·5% of the total. Of course, a very large number of these were in use for long-stay patients. If the number of long-stay beds (i.e. those occupied by the same patient for two or more years) is deducted, we find the psychiatric units had 1,182 short-stay beds (36·1% of the total), while the mental hospitals had 2,092 such beds (63·9%). Thus, although in 1962 the mental hospitals still had about two-thirds of the short- and medium-stay hospital beds in the Region, they only dealt with 40% of new in-patient admissions, whereas the general hospital psychiatric units, with only one-third of the beds, took nearly 60%. These figures are surely startling and make nonsense of the remark that the general hospital psychiatric unit 'provides a valuable means of treating some patients, but is unsuitable for the majority' (Jones, 1961).

Figure 2 shows a small map of the area administered by the Manchester Regional Hospital Board. It indicates two of the psychiatric units and their respective catchment areas. We chose for our investigation these two out of the then seventeen existing units, because although they both had come into operation about the same time, their catchment areas had somewhat different social and economic characteristics; further, in the one case (the Burnley General Hospital unit) there were 0·4 beds per 1,000 population, while in the other (the unit linked with the Victoria General Hospital, Blackpool) there were 0·15 beds per 1,000 population. In both areas the consultant offered a very satisfactory psychiatric service, but in the one area he was completely identified with the new developments and could be described as an enthusiast, while in the other the psychiatrist

FIG. 2

THE MANCHESTER REGION

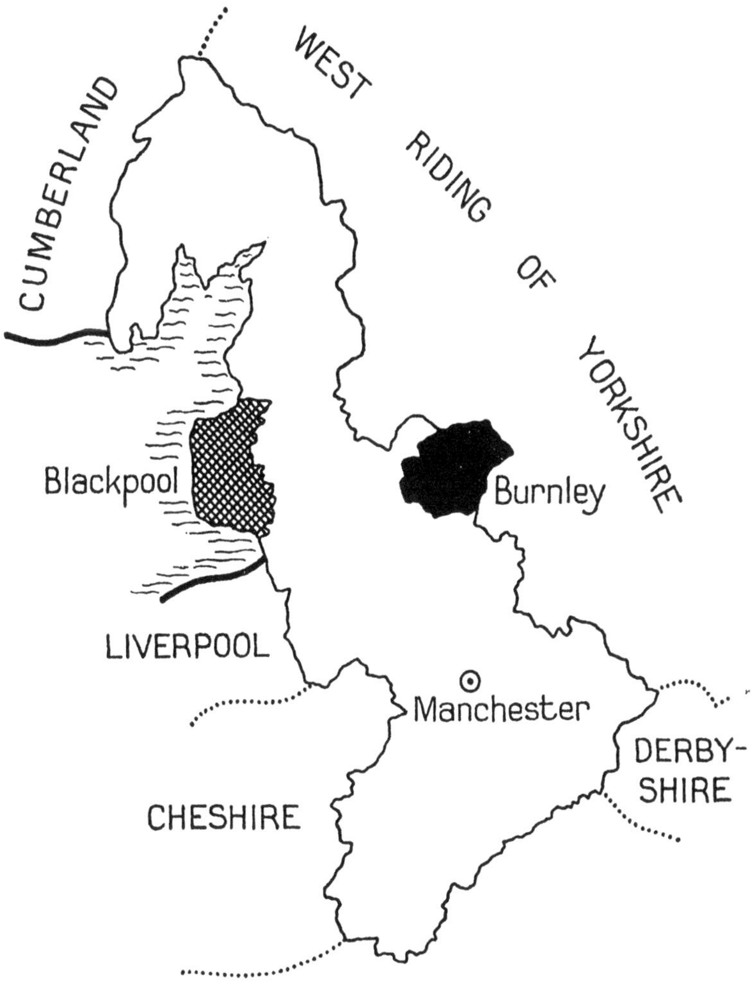

The shaded parts represent the catchment areas of the two units.

in charge expressed forcibly a number of reservations. It was thought that any differences in our respective findings might at least in part be related to any or all of the above factors. In the following chapter the two selected units and their catchment areas are severally described by their consultant psychiatrists, each of whom had been in charge from the time the units were established to that of the present investigation.

CHAPTER II

Description of Units

THE BURNLEY UNIT AND ITS CATCHMENT AREA

The development of this local psychiatric service in Burnley has undoubtedly been of benefit in terms of earlier diagnosis and treatment, quicker return to work, and reduced economic hardship in respect of the patients and families concerned. There has been a definite improvement in the community's attitudes towards the mentally ill and an increasing tendency to use the services locally available. Initially the medical, social, and geographic circumstances were all in favour of some such development. The existing psychiatric service was minimal, social provision lagged behind the times, and the nearest large mental hospital was twenty-six miles away. Yet the speedy use of the new unit when established, the co-operative attitude of the general practitioners, the high reliability rate of their referrals in terms of psychiatric need, and the acceptance of the new unit as an integral part of the general hospital service suggest that this particular community was ready to accept the new concept. No pressures were exerted by the general hospital administration or by the medical or surgical colleagues to keep 'these patients' away nor was any serious objection advanced to the special requests made, in terms of upgrading the existing facilities and staff. Other medical specialities with equally pressing needs recognized the needs of the psychiatric patients and the former neglect from which they suffered.

The following paragraphs briefly describe the catchment area, survey the history of this new service, the psychiatric unit and its working relationships and approach. Finally, points of difficulty which need special consideration for the future are indicated.

The Catchment Area

In the period under study (1958–63) the psychiatric unit was serving an area which consisted of the County Borough of Burnley and the surrounding Division (No. 6) of Lancashire County Council. The total area covered approximately 100 square miles, with a population of about 172,000 (80,500 in the County Borough, 91,240 in the County Division). The latter includes the municipal boroughs of Nelson and Colne, the urban districts of Barrowford, Brierfield, Padiham, and Trawden, and the rural district of Burnley.

The area is situated in the hilly north-east corner of Lancashire, bordering the West Riding of Yorkshire on the northern and eastern reaches; Pendle Hill (1,800 feet) forms a natural western boundary. To the south, the road and rail communications in the broadening valley link the district with other industrial parts of east Lancashire.

Industry predominates along the valleys of the Calder, Brun, and Pendle Water, and small industrial sites are found in the vicinity of many hillside villages. There are small areas of arable land, while deciduous and coniferous woodlands exist around Read, Simonstone, and the Forest of Pendle, but, in general, moorland, heath and rough pasture predominate in the upland country.

At the time of survey, the chief industries were cotton, rayon, and silk manufacture, electrical and mechanical light engineering, leather tanning, textile bleaching, and dyeing. There was a small amount of deep and opencast coal-mining, and in recent years, as part of the North-east Lancashire Development Area, some new industries have been established in the district, adding new variety to employment possibilities. Thus in Burnley itself, which was once the largest weaving town in the world, dependent almost entirely on the textile trade, far more workers are to be found now in light engineering than in textiles.

In general the people are shrewd, honest, hardworking, reliable, and money-conscious; they display pride in their homes, the standard of which is relatively high. The society has tended to be 'matriarchal'; the women, more independent than average, have a long heritage of wage-earning and a strong sense of equality. They tend to control and run the home, accepting and budgeting the combined wage-packets and giving the husbands their pocket-money. These traditions have possibly contributed to the emergent fact that many women run their own businesses and take an active part in local government affairs. There is a general tendency to rigidity and anxious carefulness in the population, a reaction perhaps to the distinct insecurity of thirty or more years ago and characteristic of populations that have suffered from industrial hard times.

In 1959, when the research sample of patients was drawn, the area as a whole appeared vigorous, prosperous, and ambitious, but it was still finding it difficult to hold the younger people, with a consequent drift away on their part and thus a proportionately larger number of older people remained.

History of the Psychiatric Unit

Until November, 1956, psychiatric bed accommodation at Burnley General Hospital consisted of a closed, mainly custodial unit. There had been little or no active treatment available locally until 1955, when a psychiatric registrar, part-time social worker, and part-time secretary were appointed to assist the visiting consultant, who attended for one or two sessions weekly. It was common for direct admissions to be made to one or other of two mental hospitals, both a considerable distance away from the area; otherwise cases were lodged in the Burnley unit until transfer to these hospitals could be accepted. The visiting consultant also had sessions in other peripheral areas and at one of the mental hospitals. The average number of patients admitted monthly under this régime amounted to twelve to fourteen, with an equal distribution of the sexes. Out-patient attendances at one or two clinics a week were usually in single figures.

On the locked and barred wards of the unit, darkly painted and using direct-current lighting, seclusion and restraint were still employed; knives, forks, razors, and mirrors were not allowed and the staff were definitely custodial in their attitudes.

In November, 1956, a part-time consultant was appointed to the unit, a medical secretary, and a doubly-trained sister. A new informal female ward was opened and the psychiatric department raised, centralized, and controlled its own case-sheets and ran its own appointment system. Very shortly a part-time psychiatric social worker was appointed to the unit and a senior house officer. The medical staffing then consisted of one part-time consultant (at least six sessions to the hospital group), one registrar, and one senior house officer – a basic staffing structure which was still in being at the time of the research survey.

In the first six months, as these various changes took place, increasing use was made of the psychiatric services. A local branch of the National Association of Mental Health was formed, a psychiatric social club opened, two further mental welfare officers appointed by the local authority, a Mental Health Exhibition was shown at the hospital, and in May, 1957, the seclusion register was finally closed. After twenty months the upgrading of the female block was completed and informal patients were able to be admitted on the male side, where upgrading was finally completed in August, 1959. In April of that year the last unit patient was 'decertified' under the old legislation and no long-term compulsory detention has been required since.

TABLE I

Breakdown of transfers to major mental hospitals from August to September annually

The Burnley Unit

	Male		*Female*		
	Vol.	*Cert.*	*Vol.*	*Cert.*	*Totals*
1951	4	27	1	27	59
1952	3	22	1	19	45
1953	5	19	5	17	46
1954	4	13	2	12	31
1955	2	12	2	20	36
1956	2	6	0	11	19
1957	0	3	0	4	7
1958	0	3	1	2	6
1959	0	0	2	0	2
1960	0	0	0	0	0
1961	0	0	1	0	1
1962	2	0	3	0	5
1963	3	0	1	0	4

Attendance and admission rates reflected the increasing use of the new psychiatric unit. Thus, by October, 1958, within twelve months, fifty-five active beds were receiving and discharging voluntary and informal patients; there were nearly 400 admissions and discharges in the year and over 600 new case-sheets had been raised. The changes affecting the legal status of patients admitted to the new unit is shown in the marked reduction of transfers to the major mental hospitals.

Initially the consultant spent two of his eight sessions visiting the mental hospital. Apart from accepting nominal responsibility for certain wards there and seeing occasional problem cases, the main work was found to be liaison with the staff and seeking out such cases as remained who had been admitted originally from the Burnley area. The object was to return these patients gradually to the care of the general hospital unit, then home. Once this was finished it was found that more sessional time was required in the general hospital unit, and eventually these visits to the mental hospital ceased. Good bonds, however, had been forged for future co-operation when necessary.

The Psychiatric Unit, 1959–63

During the period under survey the unit was established with a maximum of eighty active beds (0·4 beds per 1,000 population). The basic medical staff structure continued as one part-time consultant, one registrar, and one senior house officer. To this were added two general practitioners as clinical assistants in 1959. On the nursing side, in addition to one double-trained sister, three other sisters, and three charge nurses, the unit acquired a deputy matron of its own in 1960. The part-time psychiatric social worker was mainly concerned with children and adolescents, but the general social work aspect was strengthened by the appointment in the same year of a further two mental welfare officers to the local authority staff (making six in all), with whom the unit worked in close conjunction. Secretarial staff was increased by the appointment of a receptionist and assistant secretary.

The unit buildings consisted of one male and one female hospital block, with the addition in 1960 of a new psychiatric out-patient and treatment department, all within the curtilage of Burnley General Hospital. Supporting facilities consisted of a day-care service for senile patients (1959), a hospital industrial workshop and rehabilitation unit, to which the day-care service was transferred (1961), enlarged local authority sheltered workshop accommodation (1960), and a half-way hostel for sixteen male or female ex-patients (1962). The psychiatric social club remained active, its programme bringing many local organizations into contact with mentally ill patients and doing much to modify public attitudes. In 1963 the local Alcoholics Anonymous group were linked with the hospital rehabilitation unit, and weekly meetings were established.

Since the survey ended in 1963, the following developments have taken place: Further amendments were made to the medical staff structure, leading to the present establishment of one part-time consultant (eight sessions), one medical assistant, two registrars and two general practitioners (clinical assistants), giving two sessions a week each. The establishment for a clinical psychologist has not yet been filled, nor that for a workshop supervisor. The nursing establishment continues to be well below strength, and it seems probable that in future more reliance will need to be placed upon State-enrolled and pupil nurses, when the unit eventually accepts responsibility for their training. The number of treatment sessions has been increased. Group therapy in small closed groups, conducted with a dynamic orientation, has begun in the evenings. Cookery, dressmaking classes, ward occupational therapy, and art therapy have been developed. In the male block a mixed ward for both male and female patients was opened in 1964. In the same year a pilot trial was begun of the use of L.S.D. as an aid to psychotherapy in the treatment of personality disorder and severe phobic and obsessional states.

The Work of the Psychiatric Unit

The psychiatric unit by its own example and methods of work influences the other specialities and departments in the hospital. Psychiatry has also much to offer in terms of human relations and an understanding of emotional factors in disease to her sister specialities. Any steps which bring psychiatry and psychiatrists' views to the general body of medical thoughts and actions must be regarded as healthy and normal ones. The close links established with consultant colleagues (and indeed with general practitioners) have undoubtedly inspired confidence in the ability of psychiatry to offer something to the patient. This leads to earlier diagnosis and treatment, and with this a reduction in frequency of cases requiring compulsory admission or in states of severely disturbed behaviour.

The unit in its turn has derived benefit from the proximity of the general hospital. Both medical and nursing staff are less divorced from general medicine and so are more aware and interested in the general organic problems of medicine and surgery and more capable of managing them. Special medical care is also more easily organized in this general hospital *milieu*; for example, cases of neurosis with presenting physical symptoms and psychosomatic disorders are more readily seen, arrangements for screening and treatment of attempted suicides are facilitated, and so on.

Since the unit is accessible and open to the community, both lay and professional, this allays fear, prejudice, and doubt and encourages individual interest and confidence. Personalities are involved rather than paper references. Far fewer local authorities are dealt with than by the large mental hospitals. Day-to-day contacts between unit, general practitioner, and local authority staff promote appreciation of each other's contributions and problems. Early reference, pre-clinic screening, social care, and follow-up visits have more impact and meaning within the framework of the total community team. The individual with his individual disorder and problems remains more easily an individual where opportunities are present for special problems to be considered at a realistic case-conference level with all associated workers present. Decisions are then more likely to be implemented and can be more readily checked.

Two diagnostic clinics – one at night – are held weekly, when the consultant sees all new out-patients and a programme of treatment is planned. The unit policy is to begin and continue intensive treatment as soon as patients are accepted and a case-sheet raised. The aim is to arrange this for the individual, involving the family and community whenever necessary, but in general attempting to make him accept his responsibilities both at home and at work, whilst treatment continues. Initial admissions are freely used to enhance this aim. Delays in treatment are initial ones, produced by the waiting period between actual paper referral and the time when the patient attends the clinic; this is usually five to six weeks. If a case is more urgent than would initially appear or be known, pre-clinical screening by mental welfare officers, domiciliary visiting, and occasionally compulsory procedures are available. Over a period of ten years (1956–66) no case from the catchment area has been refused treatment or diverted to another psychiatric hospital, and of 6,696 cases only thirty-three have been so transferred at any time. The domiciliary service does not seem to be abused, and is used for elderly patients, acute cases fearful of hospital, and patients who refuse to attend as out-patients, usually because of ignorance and prejudice which are quickly overcome.

As to the patient himself, in the small district unit the doctor–patient relationship is enhanced and more consistent. Contact with the unit through normal out-patient referral seems to encourage the acceptance of advice, treatment, and if necessary admission. Useful and successful therapy begets confidence, which is soon spread locally, the unit earning whatever reputation it obtains. In this small, compact unit, moreover, staff team-work is also enhanced and a greater uniformity of aim can be engendered in both staff and patients by the clinical director within this narrower compass. Visiting by relatives is much easier and is made at the same time as in the general hospital – daily. Access of patients and relatives to senior nursing and medical staff is purposely encouraged and seldom abused. It is possible to encourage patients to make contact and live in the normal environment of their home and town; it is also possible to encourage the community to give special consideration to the needs of psychiatric patients, so that they can continue to have access to their usual environment and habitat. To this end it is essential that there should be adequate social services – for example, home helps, night-sitters, day-centres, hostel accommodation, etc.

Problems that arise

The argument has been put forward that the claims of general hospital psychiatric units to accept and treat perfectly adequately all types of patients cannot be substantiated. The annual intake of patients at the unit, however, shows that the distributions of sex, age, and type of psychiatric disorder are comparable with accepted figures. Experience has shown that treatment can continue on a local basis provided that staff and accommodation at the unit can be maintained at a certain level and there is a close working partnership with the supporting local social services.

The major difficulties that have been found to arise centre round the necessity for security in some cases, for compulsory detention of disorderly and dangerous patients and for the prevention of an accumulation of chronic patients in the unit beds.

The unit has no facilities for restraint or strict custodial care, so that certain cases referred by the courts are not acceptable. In addition, because of the relative smallness and intimacy of these units, the occasional disturbing or dangerous case may require transfer to a mental hospital. But the number so transferred has proved negligible over the years, and it is rare that the difficult epileptic or psychopath has become too much of a problem for the unit staff or that the half-hearted alcoholic has outworn his welcome. As mentioned above, the last patient to be legally 'certified' in the unit was at the beginning of 1959.

The problem of an accumulation of chronic patients in the unit beds has been carefully watched over the years. In 1957 the original chronic population numbered sixty-five patients (thirty-seven female, twenty-eight male); in the subsequent seven years there was a certain amount of movement and seventy-four chronic patients were newly admitted (thirty-nine female, thirty-five male). At present (1964) the chronic population number thirty-eight patients (twenty-two female, sixteen male). It would seem therefore that the use of geriatric services (hospital and domiciliary), hostel accommodation, and the natural processes of death do much to prevent the expected silting up of accommodation in these small psychiatric units. That there was no transfer of the load to the distant mental hospitals is shown by the fact that over seven years only four chronic patients were so accommodated, and in turn six such patients were received from the mental hospital by the unit for care and resettlement in their own community.

Closely allied with the question of chronicity and the whole policy of early admission and discharge back into the community is the frequency of the readmission rate. This relates in particular to the small number of patients who might well once have become long-term admissions. Good staff attitudes towards the recurring problems help during the periods of remission and maintain the level of behaviour in the community, while mutual trust between community and unit leads to earlier readmission and less deterioration. Increasing interest and support from the local authority mental welfare officers has been of great assistance and the presence of the sheltered workshop and hostel latterly a great asset, especially for the schizophrenic patients. The unit's own workshop and rehabilitation centre has an average attendance of forty-five patients daily and the associated senile dementia day-care service has a register of some thirty-three patients (an average of sixteen patients daily). A closer follow-up of readmissions, when more than three have occurred, has been planned; this will involve regular three-monthly clinic appointments and monthly visits by the mental welfare officers, to see whether readmissions can be reduced in frequency or in length of stay.

In conclusion, it may be said that there would not seem to be any right point or advantage in perpetuating the segregation and isolation of patients from their community because they are mentally ill or for some reasons of economic, parochial, or political expediency. It is true that needs will have to be assessed according to local conditions. In large cities the answer may lie in sectorization, with the equivalent of a district general hospital, such as Burnley, providing for most of the medical (including psychiatric) needs of a population of some 150,000 to 200,000. This is not to preclude regional experiments for the development of special units to investigate the treatment of schizophrenia, for example, or psychopathic states, as aids to the more general type of unit. In rural areas with scattered populations one general hospital psychiatric unit may have to be complemented by smaller day hospital units with perhaps a few emergency beds. However that may be, there is no doubt that in an area such as we have described above there is good evidence now to show that a general hospital psychiatric unit can indeed meet the main psychiatric needs of the population with a ratio of 0·4 beds per 1,000 persons. There must also be adequate geriatric services and social services in the hospital and the community, with realistic co-operation among the personalities involved in their management and daily functioning.

E. T. Downham, M.D., M.B., C.L.B., D.P.M.,
Consultant Psychiatrist,
Burnley and District Hospital Management Committee.

THE BLACKPOOL UNIT AND ITS CATCHMENT AREA

In this Region – that is, the area administered by the Manchester Regional Hospital Board – the policy for psychiatric units in a general hospital is clearly known to all as predominantly an out-patient policy. Professional freedom was never, of course, threatened in any way whatsoever, but there were numerous implicit pressures against admitting patients to in-patient status, or if patients were so admitted, the time of sojourn was expected to be no more than a minimum. Circulation of statistical returns from all units in the Region kept a competitive spirit alive in this field. The general body of psychiatric thought in the country was developing along similar lines and the Ministry of Health actively encouraged the policy also. Thus every new patient was assessed from the point of view of out-patient treatment in the first instance, and many who appear in the records as 'admissions' were in fact those who had failed to improve after long or short out-patient experience. It seems, however, beyond doubt that individual psychiatrists will vary in the rigour with which they apply a policy of non-admission, and the writer has to admit that he had no fanatical objection to admitting patients to in-patient accommodation. If social stresses and strains occasioned by the illness were deemed to be harsh, the patient would be admitted, irrespective of the severity of the case, since psychiatric illness is judged to be very often a group or family concern (e.g. Kreitman, 1962), subtly involving some or many members. Since, too, the service was a new one for patients and general practitioners and marked a change from institutional to community care, it was thought justifiable to interpret the implicit rules with moderation in order to accrue some goodwill for the new policy as a whole. The unit, therefore, gained a somewhat unenviable reputation of being a 'heavy admitter'. But often enough it seemed that admission was justified, first of all, as a respite for both patient and family, producing an alteration of forces of an environmental nature operative in the case; in the second place, it had value as an educational and insightful experience for the patient, for, as will be shown presently, the psychiatric personnel had no time for standard psychotherapeutic conversation (Ferguson, 1961); others coming later into the field have also commented on this more recently (Le Gassicke, 1966). Nevertheless, every patient was discharged at the earliest possible moment consistent with reasonable social arrangements for his reintegration, though community organization of support not infrequently has been little more than rudimentary.

The Catchment Area

The catchment area of this psychiatric unit is the coastal strip of Lancashire, known as the Fylde. It includes the County Borough of Blackpool (*c.* 150,000 population) and Health Division 3 of Lancashire County Council (*c.* 130,000 population).

Blackpool itself is a teeming seaside resort of national, if not international, renown. In summer, at the height of the British holiday season, its population rises for a short time to astronomical heights, estimated at 1 million or thereabouts. Holiday visitors make little difference to the psychiatric unit, and only a few cases accrue in contrast with the other hospital specialities, e.g. medicine, orthopaedic surgery, etc., who are inundated and at times almost swamped by case material from holiday-makers. The endemic population of Blackpool, however, consists mainly of fairly prosperous, middle-class entrepreneurs of the holiday trade, who are augmented during the season by an influx of unskilled workers in the catering trade (Social Class V), who tend to have an uneven work record and considerable geographical mobility, though a proportion of the older ones make permanent homes in the town.

In the northern part of the area there is a fishing and trawling port. The population is mainly Social Classes IV and V, and housing conditions are rather drab and poor compared with Blackpool, and on the whole the general standard of living is lower.

In addition there are two extensive boroughs, one just north and one just south of Blackpool and contiguous with its boundaries. Their joint population is in the region of 90,000, mainly Social Classes II and III. There are many professional and business people (many of whom commute to industrial areas and use this area as a dormitory), plus a very high proportion of retired persons of some substance, who characteristically have saved up enough to buy a 'bungalow at the coast' with a view to retiring and ending their days there.

There is a rural, agricultural hinterland with a fertile soil, which is intensively cultivated; population density is low, but standards of living are characteristically comfortable.

Industry is not a feature of the district. The holiday trade enjoys pride of place and trawling has been established for many years. Imperial Chemical Industries, however, now have four or five plants in production and employ a growing number of people, while the Atomic Energy Commission Works, just outside the area, draws appreciably on the working population of that area. There is also a noteworthy representation of Civil Service departments and Governmental offices.

The living conditions are in general clearly superior to those obtaining in most of industrial Lancashire. Housing standards are on the whole high; the people are prosperous and poverty is not a feature. It is a desirable residential area, and from the medical point of view extensive private practice has always existed, and indeed still does. High standards of medical care have always been demanded, and these expectations have not, of course, been lowered by the advent of the National Health Service. There is considerable pressure on general practitioners to give a fully acceptable service, and the pressure is clearly transmitted and perceived at the hospital level.

The retirement phenomenon, previously referred to, causes the average age of the local population to rise and, since there are many 'immigrants' from east Lancashire and elsewhere, relative social isolation makes notable demands on the geriatric, psychiatric, and especially psychogeriatric services. On the whole the area is very low in social cohesiveness.

History of the Unit

Previous to the appointment of the writer as the area's first consultant psychiatrist in 1959, the psychiatric service had been a skeleton one serviced by a mental hospital some ten miles away, where there were forty-four statutory beds (observation wards), with minimal psychiatric supervision and very little treatment apart from drugs. Three established diagnostic out-patient clinics were held, two at the area general hospital and one at the local authority health centre. They were manned by a pool of psychiatrists from the mental hospital, with no key and leading figure as reference-point, exercising continuing supervision. There was also some quite extensive domiciliary visiting.

The Psychiatric Unit, 1959–63

The unit came into being just as the Mental Health Act (1959) was being drafted, and the catch-phrase 'community care' had still a good deal of evocative power; there was a general air of pioneering and near-missionary zeal inspiring the personnel in those early days.

Forty-four acute psychiatric beds (twenty-two male, twenty-two female) were made available in the wards of a geriatric hospital of 346 beds, Wesham Park Hospital. This had previously been a poor law institution and, socially speaking, some of that historical aura still adhered. However, the wards were comfortable and cheerful and they rapidly became the effective central strength of the unit. The main criticism was that the unit was situated some ten miles away from the main population centre of Blackpool. A completely new out-patient treatment centre, however, was opened on this same site. Previously there had been no *treatment* facilities for out-patients in the area. Treatment at the new centre consisted almost wholly of electro-convulsive therapy, and other procedures, such as abreaction, pentothal sleep-treatment, hypnosis, group therapy, and sundry others. Because of the distance from the main centres of population, the service depended heavily upon the availability of vehicle transport from the local authorities, and this was freely given.

Additional beds were available at the mental hospital for the catchment area (twenty-six miles away). There was ready access there to short-, medium-, long-stay, and closed wards. It was felt that this was essential to the viability of the unit, especially the closed-ward accommodation for disturbed, violent, and medico-legal cases.

Three *diagnostic* out-patient sessions were held each week, two in the general hospital and one at the local authority health centre in Blackpool. This was partly due to the shortage of room at Wesham Park and partly to the co-operation and interest of the Medical Officer of Health, who contributed greatly to the establishment of the new service by his goodwill. The mainstream of cases arose from ordinary requests for out-patient appointments by general practitioners in the area. Similarly, but to a much lesser extent, there were referrals from hospital colleagues and the occasional medico-legal case. Routine referrals quickly built up and a waiting-list of one to two months (usually the latter) became customary. Each clinic session would include one or two cases seen at short notice as a result of an urgent telephone call from a general practitioner or mental welfare officer.

There were also ward consultations in the area and other general hospitals of the group. The full spectrum of psychiatric diagnoses was encountered, but attempted suicide was by far the commonest single reason for these consultations, which averaged at six per week. Bureaucratic considerations often inspired them, owing to the house rule that 'all attempted suicides shall be seen by a psychiatrist prior to discharge'.

Domiciliary consultation was frequently requested by the general practitioners. This has obvious 'queue-jumping' advantages, but often there was no other way to deal with such cases as senile dementia, the unwilling patient, the florid psychotic. Moreover, the domiciliary visiting service had previously been utilized to cover gaps when local psychiatric organization had been sketchy, and it had acquired a functionally useful reputation. Domiciliary visits amounted to *c.* 200 to 300 a year. They constituted a heavy, time-consuming, but lucrative obligation.

As in most other branches of medicine since the inception of the National Health Service, the custom has grown up for patients to decide to have their first consultation privately and any subsequent treatment under the State service. The unit accepted 100 to 150 cases annually from this source.

During the first year of the period under review the staff consisted of one consultant psychiatrist, aided by two sessions weekly from a senior hospital medical officer from the mental hospital. A registrar was in post for two months of the year, and a general practitioner was engaged for three sessions per week as an anaesthetist at the out-patient treatment. The staff has now grown to two consultants, a registrar, plus three clinical assistant sessions, contributed by three general practitioners and some anaesthetic sessions.

The following time-table evolved:

Day	*Morning*	*Afternoon*
Monday	Unit out-patient treatment, followed by ward round	Out-patient clinic
Tuesday	Mental hospital ward visits	Private patients
Wednesday	Unit out-patient treatment, followed by ward round	Out-patient clinic
Thursday	Mental hospital ward visits	Private patients
Friday	Unit out-patient treatment, followed by ward round	Out-patient clinic
Saturday	Unit ward round and interviews with relatives	

At the unit there were forty-four acute in-patients, and, as can be seen, the equivalent of two full sessions was given to them – not a great deal of time, one might think. The diagnostic out-patient sessions were harassing and crowded occasions. There were never less than twelve and usually more than twenty patients present, and sessions extended regularly well over the allotted hours. At the mental hospital all admissions from the area were supervised and interviewed by the consultant, though treatment was usually delegated to a hospital junior medical officer. The intention was to keep in touch with the development of individual cases, so that there should be no loss of continuity on return to the parent area. This was not very popular with the administration, who regretted that highly paid personnel should spend so much time in travelling, but the medical staff remained unshaken in their confidence that the continuing doctor–patient contact was wholly desirable and well worth the sacrifice in time.

Since it is customary for all appointees to these consultant posts in psychiatric units to be given a part-time contract of nine sessions, there is tacit encouragement to engage in private practice. Such work was found to be extremely time-absorbing and demanding, and this aspect of the work eroded both the evening hours and the week-ends.

Domiciliary consultations (averaging five per week) had to be pushed in during mealtimes, in the evenings, and at week-ends. Nor does the above time-table allow for ward consultations, which were regularly requested in other departments and hospitals; nor can it indicate the constant disruptions of the programme by emergencies. Again, there was an unwritten condition that somehow it was incumbent on the consultant-in-charge to see all new cases and no patient was to be admitted to a bed unless 'vetted' in this way first. It was surprising how nearly this ideal and unattainable state of affairs was approached!

In conclusion, it is true to say that the unit enjoyed a great deal of goodwill locally, both from the hospital and the general practitioner worlds. There was a distinct feeling of local pride in the undertaking and there was an intimacy with colleagues produced by the closed nature of the area, that undoubtedly made working conditions more agreeable. First names were regularly used by fellow consultants and general practitioners, and this informality was achieved through contacts over meals at the area general hospital and through the active medical social life of the district. Most of the other branches of medicine and most general practitioners fully appreciated the scope and limitations of this new approach to treatment of the mentally ill.

It seems, from the follow-up studies here reported, that the unit functioned well enough, though one had constant misgivings over what seemed to be the rushed, superficial nature of the work. All too often one felt one was offering the semblance rather than the reality of treatment, an uncomfortable state of mind to be in, unless one cynically accepts the extreme view of psychiatry as simply one of society's checks and balances. Lastly, it ought to be said that the number of hours that had to be worked (not infrequently seventy plus per week) and the unending demands for one's services gradually but inevitably made the work frankly distasteful. The attempt to reconcile Hippocratic philosophy (i.e. one cannot refuse one's services) with the preservation of the mental poise essential to the discharge of obligations to patients under care, was almost the most difficult single exercise in the undertaking. In the short run, relatively speaking, the patients appear to have done well enough. In the long run, however, it may be that psychiatry will be the sufferer and reassurance on this point will sooner or later become necessary.

R. S. Ferguson, M.D., D.P.M.,
Research Fellow,
Department of Sociology, Royal College of Advanced Technology, Salford.
(late Consultant Psychiatrist,
Blackpool and Fylde Hospital Management Committee).

CHAPTER III

The Investigation

INTRODUCTION

The various psychiatric units in general hospitals, which had been established over the years, seemed to work very satisfactorily and had indeed become an integral part of the mental health services of the Manchester Region. Their work was not only known from the general statistical returns submitted to the Regional Hospital Board as a matter of routine, but a number of consultants had also written surveys of their own units, which gave a descriptive account of them (Leyberg, 1959; Freeman, 1960; Silverman, 1961). These descriptions drew a vivid picture of the work as it presented itself to those who were occupied in it. This, however, was not necessarily the complete picture. It only reported on those patients who actually came to the units or returned there when they fell ill again. It could not throw much light on those who failed to return. Did they seek treatment elsewhere? Nor could assessments be made as to how large a number of patients living in the community engaged other services. Did they swell the work of the general practitioners or strain the existing social services? These questions were difficult to answer and in fact require special planned investigation. Most of all there was a nagging doubt as to what this new kind of management of psychiatric patients might mean for their families. So far no systematic investigations had been made into what kind of burden was devolving on the patients' households, or to what extent their position might have been eased by this new type of management, as compared with what occurs in the more conventional kind of service.

These questions had, of course, never been overlooked or forgotten by the doctors who ran these psychiatric units; indeed, some of them were much concerned. Therefore, when the University Department of Psychiatry suggested a systematic investigation which would throw light precisely on these aspects, the suggestion was taken up at once by the Mental Health Subcommittee of the Regional Hospital Board, who welcomed a thorough inquiry by an independent observer and very willingly and generously provided a grant towards the financing of such an investigation. The actual plan of this was left entirely to the University research team, and the Regional Hospital Board did not in any way try to influence the inquiry, although remaining most helpful throughout in providing the necessary documents and obtaining permission from the hospital authorities for the work to be carried out.

The questions we wanted to ask were, first of all, do these psychiatric units really achieve what they set out to do – namely, to look after an unselected group of psychiatric patients effectively without recourse to long-term hospitalization, in particular long-term mental hospitalization? Secondly, how do the patients themselves fare under such management? We wanted to know how it affects their clinical condition and their social adjustment – in particular, their work record. Thirdly, we wanted to know to what extent the patients engage medical and social services other than those of the unit itself, and, fourthly, what kind of burden does this largely extramural management devolve on the patients' households? Finally, we wanted to carry out what might be called 'consumer research' – an attempt to find out what patients and relatives feel about their experience of the new service.

In order to answer the above questions, we needed to know exactly how the patients had fared during a given period (we chose a period of four years) after they had first been seen at the psychiatric unit. Our study, therefore, consisted of a four-year follow-up of patients newly incepted by the units in the course of one year. The follow-up was carried out by one research psychiatric social worker, who did the fieldwork of contacting and interviewing patients and relatives in the two catchment areas. The general aim was to obtain an account of what effect this type of management had on the patients, on the services, and on the households, and to find in particular if any special difficulties had arisen. We set out to find if there were any weaknesses of the new system and if possible some indications of their cause, so that suggestions might emerge for their elimination.

METHOD

(*a*) *The Sample*

The actual investigation was started in June, 1962. We began by obtaining a representative sample of new patients seen in each of the two selected units over a twelve-month period. Each unit, though responsible for a certain catchment area, did see a number of patients who lived outside that area. For obvious reasons, such patients were not turned away, and not only took up out-patient appointments but also in-patient or day-patient space. Their numbers were not necessarily trivial; for instance, in the Burnley unit 155 patients out of 711 first inceptions resided outside the catchment area in the year under review. This is a point worth keeping in mind when the minimum requirements for services of this type are being discussed. For the purpose of the present investigation, we confined ourselves to those patients residing *within the catchment area.* This allowed us to relate our findings to a definite population about which comparable sociological data could be obtained.

We further confined ourselves to *first* admissions to the service, but eliminated patients under the age of sixteen years, and also persons seen solely for National Service examinations, etc.

We then listed all those first admissions over the age of sixteen years who resided in the catchment areas and who had attended the units for the first time during the period 1 November 1958–31 October 1959, in the case of the Burnley unit, and 1 May 1959–30 April 1960, in the case of the Blackpool unit. Although only first referrals to the units were included in our sample, this was irrespective of the previous length of illness or whether the patients had been treated elsewhere before coming to the unit. It was also irrespective of whether the patients were incepted as out-patients (which the majority were), or whether they were seen on a domiciliary visit or had come directly into the unit as in-patients, or were first seen by way of consultation while in-patients in another hospital ward, e.g. medical, surgical, or obstetric.

TABLE 2

Stratification of research sample

	Density of Sample	Blackpool		Burnley		Total	
		Clinic Total	*Sample*	*Clinic Total*	*Sample*	*Clinic Total*	*Samples*
Over 60							
All diagnoses	50%	84	42	94	47	178	89
Under 60							
Organic psychosyndrome	100%	9	9	4	4	13	13
Schizophrenia	100%	41	41	17	17	58	58
Epilepsy	100%	5	5	5	5	10	10
All other diagnoses	16–13%	357	56	343	47	700	103
All ages	31–25%	496	153	463	120	959	273

Our list comprised, therefore, the entire intake for a twelve-month period of new patients defined in the terms mentioned above. The totals amounted to 463 patients for the Burnley unit and 496 patients for the Blackpool unit, a final total of 959 patients. Since our inquiry was intended to be thorough and detailed, but had to be encompassed by only one field-worker, a representative sample was then drawn from this large group of patients. The results are shown in Table 2.

We decided not to take a straightforward random sample, but a stratified one, so that those patients who were likely to present more serious problems to the service would be represented more densely in the sample. The vulnerable groups were considered to be the elderly (over sixty years) and certain diagnostic groups, such as the organic psychosyndromes, epilepsies, and schizophrenias, all of which illnesses tend to run a very chronic course and in the past have required long hospitalization for large numbers of patients.

We therefore divided the total list of 959 patients into those who were over and those who were under sixty years of age, and selected every other patient over sixty years, thus giving a 50% sample of older patients. Of those under sixty years of age, we selected all those who fell into the three vulnerable diagnostic groups named above, and included every one of them in the sample (100%). Of the remaining diagnostic groups we took a 13% sample from the Burnley unit and a 16% sample in the

TABLE 3

Diagnostic composition of research sample

Diagnosis	*Blackpool*		*Burnley*		*Total*	
Organic psychosyndrome	22	14·4%	14	11·7%	36	13·2%
Schizophrenia	44	28·8%	18	15%	62	22·7%
Affective psychosis	34	22·3%	34	28·3%	68	25%
Epilepsy	5	3·3%	5	4·2%	10	3·6%
Personality disorder	31	20·2%	38	31·7%	69	25·3%
Abnormal psychogenic reaction	14	9·1%	8	6·7%	22	8·0%
Other	3	1·9%	3	2·4%	6	2·2%
	153	100%	120	100%	273	100%

case of the Blackpool unit. The individual diagnoses had been made by the two consultants in charge of the respective units, and were grouped into the aetiological classification illustrated in Table 3.

This stratification of the sample should be borne in mind when appraising the results, because the stratification in itself will tend to magnify difficulties, due to the loading of the research sample with the most problematic group of patients.

(*b*) *The Follow-up*

It was planned to carry out a four-year follow-up study on the selected sample, treating the group of patients as a cohort and obtaining information which would relate not only to the final outcome (cross-sectional view), but to what had occurred throughout the period as a whole (longitudinal view).

As our research instrument we used a coded item sheet.[1] This was filled in by the research field-worker following semi-structured interviews both with the patient and a member of the household where practicable. The information thus gained was coded in such a way that it then lent itself to Hollerith analysis. The field-worker endeavoured to see every member of the cohort and a household member personally, usually by means of a home visit, when an attempt would be made to interview patient and other informants separately. The interview was planned to fall approximately four years after the patient had first been incepted into the service. Each interview was to take approximately one and a half to two hours. In addition, full use was made of records, both hospital and other. Before the research worker visited in each case, a letter had been written, signed by the consultant in charge of the unit, introducing the field-worker to the patient and the household.

[1] When the item sheet was composed, care was taken to make the items comparable to similar investigations elsewhere, although they could not be completely identical. In particular, questionnaires used by Susser and Stein and Sainsbury and Grad (1962) were taken into account. Adjustments had to be made, as none of these workers was concerned with retrospective studies. We would like to take the opportunity of expressing our gratitude for their help and co-operation.

(*c*) *The Results*

A great deal of co-operation was obtained from the patients and their families but, owing to deaths, removals, refusals, and sometimes inadequate records, it was not possible to obtain answers to every question on the schedule in every case. Nevertheless, some information was elicited about every single patient in the sample. On account of these variations in the basic data, totals in the different sections of the inquiry will be found to differ at times, and this should be related to the above facts.

In 115 cases (sixty-two in the Blackpool unit, fifty-three in the Burnley unit) both the patient and the relative could be interviewed.

In forty-seven cases (twenty-four in the Blackpool unit, twenty-three in the Burnley unit) only the patient could be interviewed.

In seventy-six cases (forty-one in the Blackpool unit, thirty-five in the Burnley unit) only the informant could be interviewed.

In the remaining thirty-five cases (twenty-six in the Blackpool unit, nine in the Burnley unit) information could only be gleaned from records and in some cases by letter from relatives overseas.

The high figure of untraceable cases in Blackpool reflects the greater mobility of the population in that area and it presented us with something of a problem. Every effort was made to contact, and a considerable amount of valuable time was expended in this direction.

It must be borne in mind that the patients to be followed up were often not the ordinary in-patient population, but patients seen briefly at out-patient clinics, who had never come to form any regular relationship with the units. Because of this sometimes tenuous relationship with the units over the four years and because of the specific difficulties that are apt to arise when problems of a psychiatric nature are under investigation, skilled interviewing was called for, and we were fortunate to obtain the services of a professional psychiatric social worker for the task.

TABLE 4

Sex composition and clinic usage

	BLACKPOOL				BURNLEY				BOTH UNITS			
	Population over 16 years (Census 1961)	*Clinic population*	*Research sample*	*Clinic usage per 10,000 population*	*Population over 16 years (Census 1961)*	*Clinic population*	*Research sample*	*Clinic usage per 10,000 population*	*Population over 16 years (Census 1961)*	*Clinic population*	*Research sample*	*Clinic usage per 10,000 population*
Male	133,926 47%	209 42%	75 49%	16	73,718 47%	189 41%	43 36%	26	207,644 47%	398 42%	118 43%	19
Female	153,420 53%	287 58%	78 51%	18	82,062 53%	274 59%	77 64%	33	235,482 53%	561 58%	155 57%	24
Both sexes	287,346 100%	496 100%	153 100%	17	155,780 100%	463 100%	120 100%	30	443,126 100%	959 100%	273 100%	22

FINDINGS

(a) *Descriptive Data on Sample*

The following sections will give an analysis of the findings in the entire sample, i.e. in the total group of 273 patients from both units. This seems a legitimate way of analysing our results in view of the far-reaching similarities between the two sets of data. Wherever differences do arise, however, we shall make a point of drawing attention to them and examine them, where possible, to find the reasons for such differences or any likely effects these may have had on the outcome.

Table 4 shows the sex distribution in the general population of the catchment area, in the clinic population, and in the research sample for the two units separately and together. It can be seen that the sex distribution in the general population of the catchment areas is identical (47% men, 53% women). In the clinic populations, the women are over-represented, and this applies to both the Blackpool and the Burnley unit, but the difference is only small – namely, 5%. The question that arises is: Why do the research samples in the two units show a different sex distribution? It seems that in Blackpool the men and in Burnley the women are over-represented. To explain this it should be noted that the usage of the units per 10,000 population also differs in the two areas and is very significantly higher in Burnley – in fact, almost double that in the Blackpool area. In the Blackpool area only seventeen per 10,000 population, in Burnley thirty per 10,000 population are seen at the unit ($p < 0{\cdot}001$). The difference in clinic usage seems largely accounted for (though not entirely so) by more women being referred to the Burnley unit. They are clearly over-represented and account for much of the excess usage in the sample.

Another factor also accounts for the sex difference in the two research samples. It appears that different diagnostic groups used the units in different ratios. Whereas the ratio of schizophrenic patients per 10,000 population is the same in the two units, we found that the other diagnostic categories were not as frequent in Blackpool as in Burnley. In other words, whereas there seemed to be some reluctance in the Blackpool catchment area to make use of the psychiatric unit as compared with Burnley, this reluctance seemed overcome in the case of schizophrenic patients, who turned up in the same ratio in both units. This seems to suggest that the number of newly incepted schizophrenics in the two units were more closely related to the incidence of this illness in the two populations than were the other diagnostic groups, always assuming that they had a similar incidence in both populations, but in their case this was not reflected in the attendance at the units. Schizophrenia is such a conspicuous and frightening disease that the social pressures which tend to keep patients away from the clinic were brushed aside (Hare, 1955).

Since we used a stratified sample for our research purpose, in which the diagnosis of schizophrenia was a factor, this will also account for certain differences in the sex and age distribution in the two samples. As shown in Table 14, the Blackpool sample contained many more schizophrenics than did the Burnley sample. Since most of these were young males, the Blackpool sample as a whole contained a higher proportion of male patients (49%), whereas in Burnley the figure was 36%. It will be seen that there was also a difference in the age-composition. The point is clinched if the number of schizophrenics in the Blackpool sample is brought down to the same level as that found in the Burnley sample. The difference in sex distribution, and age for that matter, between the two research samples then disappears. It can be reasonably assumed that these differences are due to the relative over-representation of schizophrenics in the Blackpool sample, or, more correctly speaking, to the relative under-representation of the other diagnostic groups brought about by the smaller clinic usage in the Blackpool area.

It is clear, therefore, that certain artefacts have entered here, and the findings in the research sample cannot all be related directly to the general population of the catchment area. Our main concern in this investigation, however, was to see how the two psychiatric units coped with the patients they did receive. Much of the future analysis, therefore, will have to confine itself to this purpose alone, having to forgo the otherwise desirable procedure of placing these findings in the context of the catchment area population as a whole. We did, however, relate certain of our findings to the population of the catchment area, wherever this was possible.

TABLE 5

Age-groups by sex of research sample

Age in Years	*Blackpool*						*Burnley*						*Both Units*					
	Male		*Female*		*Both Sexes*		*Male*		*Female*		*Both Sexes*		*Male*		*Female*		*Both Sexes*	
15–59	59	78·5%	52	66·5%	111	73%	29	67%	44	57%	73	61%	88	74·6%	96	61·9%	184	67·4%
60–4	9	12%	7	8·9%	16	10·4%	7	163%	14	18·2%	21	17·5%	16	13·5%	21	15·5%	37	13·5%
65–9	3		8		11		3		11		14		6		19		25	
70 and over	4	9·5%	11	24·6%	15	16·6%	4	167%	8	24·8%	12	21·5%	8	11·9%	19	24·6%	27	19·1%

So far we have adduced the difference in sex and age distribution in the research samples mainly to differences in actual clinic usage. It is, of course, also feasible that these may be due to yet other factors, such as a difference in the actual incidence of the various psychiatric conditions in the two areas. We cannot exclude such a possibility, but we feel that this would be most unlikely, and our own explanation is the more obvious one – namely, a discrepancy in actual clinic usage.

Age

Table 5 shows the different age distribution in the two samples. There were more patients under sixty years of age in the Blackpool sample, where the figure is 73% as compared with 61% in the Burnley sample ($p < 0{\cdot}02$). This is in all probability due partly to the excess of young male schizophrenic patients in the Blackpool sample, but it cannot be the whole explanation, as there is a similar but smaller difference among the women patients. A number of other differences also appear in the separate age quinquennia of the 'over sixty-year' age-groups.

TABLE 6

Civil status of patients by units

	Blackpool		*Burnley*		*Both Units*	
Single	50	33%	26	22%	76	28%
Married	83	54%	77	64%	160	59%
Widowed, separated, and divorced	20	13%	17	14%	37	13%
All patients	153	100%	120	100%	273	100%

Civil Status

There was no significant difference between the two samples in this respect, though there were somewhat more single patients (33%) in the Blackpool sample compared with 22% for the Burnley sample. A large number of the married couples in the Burnley sample belonged to the older age-groups and were pensioners. This reflects fairly well the situation in the two catchment areas as a whole, but the differences are slightly exaggerated because of the above-mentioned large number of single schizophrenics in the stratified Blackpool sample.

TABLE 7

Number of persons in patient's household

No. of Persons (including Patient)	*Blackpool*		*Burnley*		*Both Units*	
1	13	9%	9	8%	22	8%
2	42	27%	46	38%	88	32%
3	39	25%	28	23%	67	25%
4 and 5	38	25%	30	25%	68	25%
More than 5	6	4%	5	4%	11	4%
Not applicable or not known	15	10%	2	2%	17	6%

Size and Type of Household

The situation regarding civil status is also shown in the number of persons in the patient's household, as illustrated in Table 7. It will be seen that there was a slightly higher proportion of patients in the Burnley sample who came from households with

TABLE 8

Type of patient's household

Living with:	*Blackpool*		*Burnley*		*Both Units*	
Parents	33	21%	18	15%	51	19%
Spouse	69	45%	77	64%	146	54%
Grown-up children	11	7%	7	5%	18	7%
Siblings or other kin	15	10%	8	7%	23	8%
Alone	12	8%	8	7%	20	7%
No fixed abode	13	9%	2	2%	15	5%
	153	100%	120	100%	273	100%

only one other person ($p < 0.05$), the majority of which consisted of the elderly married couples, indicated above. Households of other sizes were equally distributed in the two samples.

The same point is illustrated in Table 8, which gives the type of household to which the patient belonged. Here there was a higher percentage (64%) in the Burnley sample of patients living with their spouses than in the Blackpool sample (45%) ($p < 0.01$). On the other hand, the latter showed a slightly higher percentage (21%) of patients living with their parents. In the Burnley sample the figure was only 15%. This difference is probably due to the young schizophrenic who preponderated in the Blackpool sample, where we also found a higher number of patients (9%) with no fixed abode compared with 2% in the Burnley sample, a further reflection of the different social conditions in the two areas.

Geographical Mobility

There was generally a higher mobility in the Blackpool sample than in the Burnley one, as shown in Table 9. 22% changed their address during the four years though still remaining in the catchment area, whereas in the Burnley sample only 17% did so. But as regards leaving the catchment area entirely, the differences were even more marked. The figure for this in the Blackpool sample was 21%, whereas in Burnley it was only 8% ($p < 0.01$). Thus the differences between the two samples, which show that the Burnley sample was in general more settled, had more married couples, fewer people without fixed abode and fewer inclined to leave the district, are well in keeping with the conditions found in the two catchment areas as a whole, though it is true that the differences are not so very marked.

Ethnic Groupings

There was a slight trend in the Blackpool sample towards more foreign-born patients. The proportion was 18% in Blackpool and 11% in the Burnley sample. More marked differences arose, however, if one examines how many of the patients were

TABLE 9

Geographical mobility

	Inside the Catchment Area						*Out of Catchment Area*					
	Blackpool		*Burnley*		*Both Areas*		*Blackpool*		*Burnley*		*Both Areas*	
No move	104	68%	96	80%	200	73%	107	70%	106	83%	213	78%
Moved once	21	14%	14	12%	35	13%	25	16%	5	4%	30	11%
Moved twice or more	12	8%	6	5%	18	7%	8	5%	5	4%	13	5%
Not known or not applicable	16	11%	4	3%	20	7%	13	9%	4	3%	17	6%
All patients	—		—		273	100%	—		—		273	100%

indigenous to the catchment areas. These differences are shown in Table 10.

TABLE 10

Geographical mobility

	Blackpool	*Burnley*	*Both Units*
Born in catchment area	38 25%	68 57%	106 39%
Moved into catchment area:			
(*a*) Born in other parts U.K.	87 57%	38 32%	125 46%
(*b*) Foreign-born Caucasian	5 3%	3 3%	8 3%
(*c*) Foreign-born coloured	23 15%	11 8%	34 12%
	153 100%	120 100%	273 100%

In the Blackpool sample only about one-quarter of the patients were indigenous to the area (25%), whereas in the Burnley sample the proportion was over half (57%) ($p. < 0{\cdot}001$). Most of the 'immigrants', however, were from other parts of the United Kingdom.

Education

Table 11 shows three times as many patients with grammar-school education in the Blackpool sample than in the Burnley sample ($p. < 0{\cdot}05$). There was also a higher proportion of those with further education, almost in fact twice as many. The figure was 33% for the Blackpool patients as compared with 17% for the Burnley patients.

Social Class

The social-class composition of the samples was in accordance with the above differences in the educational sphere. As shown in Table 12, there were slightly more persons in Social Classes I and II in the Blackpool sample and slightly more in Social Class III in the Burnley sample, but the differences are not significant.

TABLE II

Basic and further education of patients

		Blackpool	*Burnley*	*Both Units*
Basic education:	Secondary modern school	75%	89%	81%
	Grammar school	22%	6%	15%
	Public school	2%	5%	3%
	Special school	1%	—	1%
Further education:	None	67%	83%	75%
	Apprenticed	13%	6%	10%
	Technical school	11%	7%	9%
	Professional schools, university, etc.	9%	4%	6%

TABLE 12

Social class of patients

Social Class (R.G.)	*Blackpool*		*Burnley*		*Both Units*	
I	4	3%	3	3%	7	3%
II	30	20%	16	13%	46	17%
III	63	41%	63	53%	126	46%
IV	24	16%	21	17%	45	17%
V	21	14%	12	10%	33	12%
Not known or not applicable	11	6%	5	4%	16	5%
Total	153	100%	120	100%	273	100%

If we assess the social-class drift over the four-year period, we find that there was a greater downward drift in the Blackpool sample, where the proportion was 18% of the patients as compared with 10% of the Burnley sample. Clearly, the higher the social class, the more vulnerable to the drift that menta illness may bring about.

These differences in the two samples relating to education and social class also seem in line with these factors as they existed in the catchment area population as a whole.

TABLE 13

Religion of patients

	Blackpool		*Burnley*		*Both Units*	
Church of England	106	69%	47	39%	153	56%
Nonconformist	12	8%	21	18%	33	12%
Roman Catholic	16	10%	16	13%	32	12%
Others	10	7%	10	8%	20	7%
No religion	9	6%	26	22%	35	13%

Religious Denominations

The distribution of religious denominations was in keeping with the social-class composition of the two samples. In the first place, there were a considerable number of patients who declared themselves as not belonging to any religious denomination at all, three times as many in the Burnley sample as in the Blackpool sample. In the latter, where there were more persons of higher social class, the majority adhered to the Church of England, and very few (less than half) were Nonconformist; fewer still were of no religious denomination. In the Burnley sample, however, less than half the patients belonged to the Church of England and a much larger group declared themselves as non-religious or Nonconformist. The Roman Catholic faith was more equally represented in the two samples. These differences are significant ($p. < 0{\cdot}01$).

TABLE 14

Diagnosis

	Blackpool		*Burnley*		*Both Units*	
Organic psychosyndrome	22	14%	14	12%	36	13%
Schizophrenia	44	29%	18	15%	62	23%
Affective psychosis	34	22%	34	28%	68	25%
Epilepsy	5	3%	5	4%	10	4%
Personality disorder	31	21%	38	32%	69	25%
Abnormal psychogenic reaction	14	9%	8	7%	22	8%
Other	3	2%	3	2%	6	2%

Diagnosis

The initial diagnoses do not show a random distribution in the sample. The illnesses which tend to run a chronic course and are considered particularly difficult to manage were deliberately represented more densely in the sample. Since the catchment areas differed in size, this method of stratification led to a different diagnostic composition, particularly as regards the schizophrenics. These were nearly twice as many in the Blackpool sample. On the other hand, the differences between the two samples as regards the other diagnoses were not great at all, particularly if the personality disorders and the abnormal psychogenic reactions are taken together. In the Blackpool sample these amounted to 30%, compared with 39% in the Burnley sample.

It must not be forgotten that due to this method of stratified sampling the difficulties encountered in the management of these patients in this largely extramural setting will appear at their severest.

Furthermore, the illnesses from which the patients were suffering at inception were by no means all of recent onset. It is true that only patients that had been newly incepted by the units were included in our samples, but many had been ill for a considerable time before they appeared at the units.

TABLE 15

Duration of psychiatric illness before inception

	Blackpool		*Burnley*		*Total*	
1 month	4	2·6%	8	6·7%	12	4·5%
2–6 months	39	25·5%	29	24%	68	24·9%
7–24 months	36	23·5%	39	32·5%	75	27·5%
25 months and over	67	43·7%	41	34·2%	108	39·5%
Not known	7	4·7%	3	2·6%	10	3·6%

Table 15 shows that nearly 40% had been ill for more than two years before inception and another 27·5% had been ill for seven months to two years; the chronicity was slightly more severe in the Blackpool sample, though the difference is not statistically significant.

It should be particularly mentioned that in the case of the personality disorders, which by definition are lifelong abnormalities, 'duration of illness' has been understood in the sense of the duration of the particular crisis which brought about the patient's referral.

In addition, many patients had had previous psychiatric treatment elsewhere, as might be expected for such a chronic group. This was particularly so for the Blackpool sample, where nearly three times as many patients had received previous in-patient psychiatric treatment as in the Burnley sample. This is set out in Table 16. The psychiatric illness which had led to the referral of the patient to the unit was in many cases coupled

TABLE 16

Previous psychiatric treatment

	Blackpool		*Burnley*		*Both Units*	
None or by general practitioner only	115	74%	108	90%	223	82%
Out-patient only	5	3%	2	2%	7	2%
In-patient	33	23%	10	8%	43	16%

with a co-existing, non-psychiatric illness, either at the time of referral or later on during the four-year period. 21·3% were physically ill when first referred, and another 8·8% developed some such illness in the course of the four years of the follow-up period. There was no difference in this respect between the two units.

Under the heading of non-psychiatric illness we only counted such conditions as were quite unconnected with the psychiatric disorder that had led to referral. If the patients had, for example, cerebral arteriosclerosis giving rise to an organic psychosyndrome, this was disregarded as 'non-psychiatric' illness in this particular context. Thus the total figure of 30·3% would represent a group of people who had had non-psychiatric illnesses in addition to the number suffering from organic psychosyndromes.

All the above shows that, although we were investigating a population of newly incepted patients, we were in fact dealing with a great many very chronic patients, who had at times come under previous treatment elsewhere, and in addition to their psychiatric disorder carried a considerable amount of non-psychiatric illness. This should be kept in mind when considering the results reported below.

Summary

There were certain dissimilarities in our two research samples. Firstly, in the Burnley area a larger proportion of the catchment area population used the clinic. That much we can see clearly from our own figures as compared with the population figures. The two research samples as such, however, show other differences which cannot be related to the general population of their catchment areas, because of the stratified sampling method employed. This would have been an interesting reference to make, but it was not of primary importance for our purpose. We were primarily concerned with estimating the success or otherwise of the largely extramural management of an unselected group of psychiatric patients. The sampling employed for that purpose, weighted with cases of maximum difficulty, precludes strict comparisons with the catchment-area populations in many respects. But it is still valid to draw comparisons between the two samples themselves, to see whether differences in their social or clinical characteristics affected outcome. The significant differences, however, were relatively few.

We found them to be as follows: In the Burnley sample there were more women patients and the over-sixty year age-group were over-represented. More patients belonged to larger households and more tended to live with their spouses than in other types of family setting. The Burnley sample were also on the whole more settled, showed less mobility and contained fewer foreigners among them, or persons born outside the catchment area. There was a lower level of educational attainments. There were also certain religious differences, with more persons in the Burnley sample of Nonconformist persuasion and more Anglicans in the Blackpool sample. There were more schizophrenic patients in the Blackpool sample and in general there was rather more chronicity, i.e. patients on inception tended to have been ill for longer periods than was the case with the Burnley sample. When examining the four-year findings, we kept these differences between the samples in mind, and made sure that they did not distort the picture. It is interesting, however, that on the whole the significant differences were so few.

(*b*) *Management and Treatment*

The Initial Stage

The main point of interest in the work of these units derives from their novel way of managing patients, trying to keep them out of hospital as much as possible, or, if they have to be admitted, to keep the hospital stay as short as possible. Before giving our findings regarding the success or otherwise of this policy over the four years of observation, we shall first describe the management at inception of the patient. We shall show later that this initial management can play an important role in determining success or otherwise in the further management of the patients.

Source of Referral

To show who refers patients for treatment will illustrate in what way the work of the units is anchored in the other medical and social services and what forms of co-operation are in existence. We find the picture here in both the Blackpool and Burnley samples very similar. The majority of patients (75%) were referred by their general practitioner. In a very small number (3%) the general practitioner called in the mental welfare officer to help. In 18% of the cases consultants in other specialities were the source of referral. Thus the great majority (93%) of the patients came to the psychiatrist from other doctors. The remaining 7% were referred by various social agencies, and in 2% referral came from the mental welfare officers of the local authority direct. This aspect alone illustrates to what extent psychiatric illness has become an almost exclusive medical concern. The police, magistrates, and mental welfare officers, who used to play so important a part in bringing patients to treatment, seem to have receded into the background, as they have steadily done since the Mental Treatment Act, 1930. Before that date, all admissions to mental hospitals for treatment were under judicial order. By 1933 13·2% were voluntary admissions. This proportion has risen every year until by 1948, the year of the National Health Service Act, it reached the figure of 59·2% and of 85% by 1959, when the Mental Health Act came into operation. It was one of the aims of this Act to achieve informal medical referral, and from our present investigation it seems that similar results were achieved by this type of psychiatric unit. In other services, for example the Nuffield Clinic, Plymouth (Kessel, 1966), based on a mental, not a general hospital, where a deliberate attempt was made to bring psychiatric services nearer the community, very similar trends are shown. 90% of new patients were referred by doctors and only 8% by other social agencies, but by and large where conventional mental hospital services are still operating, this result has not been achieved to the same extent, as evidenced by the fact that a fair percentage (*c.* 15–20%) are still compulsorily admitted, implying a more liberal use of the mental welfare officer.

In the general hospital psychiatric unit, at least as far as the initial steps are concerned in bringing psychiatric illness to treatment, the patient tends to approach the doctor, and it is through doctors in the main that he reaches the psychiatrist. We will have occasion to show that the picture is similar as regards subsequent management. When social agencies enter and contribute in their own important way, this is usually done under the aegis of the psychiatrist.

Mode of Inception

The next stage to examine is how in fact the patient comes into psychiatric care. Table 17 shows that over half of the patients were first seen as out-patients, slightly more in the Blackpool sample, where the percentage was 55% as compared with 46% in the Burnley sample. Well over one-third (37%) of the patients were first seen by the psychiatrist on a domiciliary visit. This latter is a relatively new kind of service and clearly plays an important part, and it is interesting to see to what extent it was being used in each of the two areas. Both consultants have commented on this in Chapter II. In the Burnley sample it was used fairly freely, affecting 41% of the patients, whereas in the Blackpool sample only 25% of the patients were incepted into the psychiatric service by this method.

About 7% of the patients were brought directly into hospital as in-patients without being seen at out-patient clinic or on domiciliary visits first. Another 7% were first seen by way of consultation while in the care of a consultant of another speciality, either as his in-patient or out-patient. This shows that the psychiatric services were called upon by other consultants, although it is difficult to say whether these services were used by them to the full.

As regards the domiciliary visits, a number of factors can be

TABLE 17

Modes of inception
(by unit, age of patient, and physical illness)

Patient first seen	Units			Age			Physical Illness	
	Blackpool	Burnley	Both Units	15–59 Years	60–4 Years	65 Years and Over	Physical Present	Illness not Present
In out-patient department	55%	46%	51%	59%	38%	30%	32%	54%
On domiciliary visit	25%	41%	32%	21%	46%	60%	37%	30%
As in-patient in the unit	7%	8%	7%	8%	8%	4%	5%	8%
On a non-psychiatric ward by consultation	9%	4%	7%	} 12%	8%	6%	16%	8%
Other	4%	1%	3%	}				

shown to have determined this choice of inception. Table 17 shows that the elderly patients were more often seen in their homes, and this became increasingly the case with advancing age. Equally, when the patient had a concomitant non-psychiatric illness, this increased the likelihood of his being seen on a domiciliary visit rather than as an out-patient at the clinic. Table 17 shows that whereas those with no physical illness were seen as out-patients in 54% of the cases and by domiciliary visit in 30%, patients who were also physically sick came as out-patients in 32% of the cases and were seen by domiciliary visit in 37%. This table refers to physical illness other than that which gave rise to the organic psychosyndrome causing the patient's inception.

It is not surprising that the same trend can be seen when the psychiatric diagnosis is taken into account. 51% of the organic psychosyndromes were seen by domiciliary visit and only 32% as out-patients. In schizophrenia, personality disorder, and abnormal psychogenic reaction, the situation was reversed. In each of these diagnostic groups well over half the patients were seen as out-patients, and only one-fifth by domiciliary visit. The affective psychoses and epilepsies fell somewhere between the above two groups, and an equal number of patients were seen as out-patients or by domiciliary visit. As regards the affective psychoses, age-factors may have entered, since many of these patients were in the upper age-groups.

Many other factors were examined by us as to the way in which they might affect this choice of inception, among them the patient's social class. We found no very significant trend here but Social Classes IV and V received proportionately fewer domiciliary visits than did Social Class III or Classes I and II.

Throughout the survey we found that it was mainly the clinical factors, such as the diagnosis, the presence of non-psychiatric illness, and old age with infirmity, which particularly influenced this mode of inception. Thus the domiciliary service is probably of very great value, bringing psychiatric attention to patients otherwise not able to reach the psychiatrist easily or willingly, which might well lead to deferment of referral and so on. The rate of domiciliary visiting seems to be much higher than appears in some other services, such as, for example, in Plymouth (Kessel, 1966), where only 16% received domiciliary visits at inception, though the type and age of patient appeared very similar. The same may be said of the service in Aberdeen, where the figure was 17·3% (Innes *et al.*, 1962).

Disposal at Inception

After the patient had been seen by the psychiatrist and his case assessed, a decision was made as to treatment and disposal, the latter largely determined by the decision on the former. We shall call this latter process 'initial disposal'. The categories of disposal that actually occurred were few and are presented in

TABLE 18

Disposal after inception

	Blackpool		*Burnley*		*Both Units*	
To mental hospital	11	7%	—		11	4%
Unit in-patient	75	49%	73	61%	148	54%
Unit day-patient	3	2%	5	4%	8	3%
Unit out-patient	58	38%	34	28%	92	34%
To general practitioner or other	6	4%	8	7%	14	5%
	153	100%	120	100%	273	100%

Table 18. Most of them are self-explanatory. The last category 'General practitioner or other' includes the following possibilities: those patients who were seen, their case discussed, and explanation given that no further psychiatric care was required; those cases where the patient, though not needing to see the psychiatrist further, would receive treatment from his general practitioner; and, finally, those patients who were offered further care of one kind or another, but refused it. This disposal occurred in only 5% of the sample, so that relatively few patients fell into that category.

In-patient admission to mental hospital as a category of disposal is of central interest to this study. It can be seen that in the Burnley sample this disposal was never used initially. In the

Blackpool sample 7% of the patients were sent to mental hospital. In terms of the policy of avoiding this, the 7% of patients appears to indicate a degree of failure; on further examination, however, it will be shown that there were special reasons for this.

Table 18 shows that in-patient admission to the psychiatric units in the general hospitals arose very frequently (54%), but there was a discrepancy between the Blackpool sample (49%) and the Burnley sample (61%). We examined the possible reasons for the discrepancy, and came to the conclusion that the difference was related to the different size of the two units. It will be remembered that the Burnley unit, although it had a smaller catchment area population, had a larger number of beds at its disposal than the Blackpool unit. In the Burnley unit the ratio was 0·4 beds per 1,000 population, whereas the Blackpool unit had only 0·15. It is true there was a smaller clinic usage of the unit in Blackpool than of the unit in Burnley, which would reduce the pressure on unit beds and make it less than it well might have been, but it must be remembered that we are only studying *first* admissions here, and a claim was being made on these beds by readmissions in the course of the on-going work. It is quite feasible that the reason for the lower rate of in-patients in the Blackpool unit was enforced by insufficient available beds rather than due to any deliberate policy. Indeed, if we add up all the initial in-patient disposals in the Blackpool sample, both to the unit and to the mental hospital, the resulting figure of 56% comes very close to the figure of 61% in the Burnley sample, although not quite reaching it. This would seem to support the view that the Blackpool unit, because it had fewer beds, could admit only a smaller number of patients and had to divert the overflow to the mental hospital, rather than the view expressed by the psychiatrist himself. Since the avowed policy was to avoid mental hospital disposal as much as possible, fewer patients were initially admitted than would have been the case if admission could have been arranged to the general hospital. Hence the smaller total of in-patient disposal in the Blackpool sample, as compared with the Burnley one. These conclusions are supported by other evidence, which will appear later (Chapter IV, iv). What emerges so far is that in order to avoid initial disposal to mental hospital a ratio of more than 0·15 beds per 1,000 population is necessary, although it would appear that not more than 0·4 beds per 1,000 population are required.

It is interesting to see how frequently patients were initially admitted as in-patients to the units; for example, in the Burnley sample about two-thirds of the patients were managed in this way. We found that this policy of liberal admission at the initial stage becomes an important factor in determining the subsequent management. It enables the psychiatrist to study the case thoroughly, and better than would be possible during a brief examination in an out-patient department. The doctor–patient relationship and the patient's relationship to the unit as a whole grows more strongly and a bond of confidence can be created more easily; the better knowledge of the case increases the confidence of the psychiatrist in his subsequent management of the patient; and, finally, the patient and the relatives get the feeling that the complaint is being taken seriously and efforts are not being spared to bring the condition under treatment. All these factors, as every practising psychiatrist will know, make it easier to manage those patients whose conditions remain chronic or show a relapsing course.

In Table 18 both day- and out-patients are given, and together amount to 37%; the fact is that few patients were sent to day hospital at this initial stage, only 3%. As explained earlier the day-hospital service at the time of the investigation was only beginning to be developed. It has grown since then and is used to a correspondingly larger degree, though its use for the support of chronic patients was already exemplified, as shown later.

Out-patient disposal was slightly more frequently used in the Blackpool unit (40%) than in the Burnley unit (32%), but the difference was not a significant one. It is probable that this is the corollary to what has been said above on the need of the Blackpool unit, through shortage of beds, to refer an overflow of patients to mental hospital instead of being able to admit to the unit itself. There might well have been a certain reluctance on the part of patients to become patients in a mental hospital, and in borderline cases this might well lead to increased initial referral to the out-patient department, attempting this management first before resorting to a mental hospital admission.

The factors which determined initial disposal, particularly in-patient disposal, were mainly clinical. It can be seen from Table 19 that there was a tendency to admit more of the older (over sixty years) age-group as in-patients. The figures here were 72%, as compared with 51% for the younger age-group. Out-patient disposal was correspondingly more frequent in the younger age-group. Further analysis of the older age-group shows that this tendency for in-patient disposal becomes more marked with advancing age. This is discussed later in Chapter IV, Sub-section iv.

The nature of the psychiatric illness also influenced the initial disposal, as can again be seen from Table 19. The organic psychosyndromes had the highest percentage of in-patient admission (72%). The affective psychoses came very close with 70%. This was probably for the purposes of electro-convulsive treatment. The other diagnostic groups were admitted as in-patients to the extent of 50–55%. What is remarkable is that on one hand there was a high percentage of in-patient admission among the personality disorders and the abnormal psychogenic reactions, and on the other hand a relatively large percentage of out-patient management in the case of the schizophrenic patients, where almost half were not admitted. This cannot be explained entirely by the small number who refused treatment (although refusals occurred more frequently in that group than in any other), and it must be attributed to a deliberate policy in the management of this type of case. The percentages were roughly the same in both units, and lend some support to this point of view. There was, however, some discrepancy between the units in the management of personality disorder and abnormal psychogenic reaction, particularly in relation to the latter. It appears that such patients were more frequently admitted as in-patients in the Burnley sample than in the Blackpool sample. It is possible they were the borderline group, where in-patient treatment seemed less imperative, and they were kept on in greater numbers as out-patients in the Blackpool unit because of the relative shortage of unit beds. One can well imagine that a patient suffering from a neurotic reaction would be more reluctant to become an in-patient if the bed offered had to be in a distant mental hospital. Social factors, such as social class, seemed to play a minor role. Not

TABLE 19

Disposal after inception by age and diagnosis

	Type of Disposal	All Patients: Both Units	Age: 15–59 Years	Age: 60 Years and Over	Diagnosis: Organic Psychosyndrome	Diagnosis: Schizophrenia	Diagnosis: Affective Psychosis	Diagnosis: Epilepsy	Diagnosis: Personality Disorder or Abnormal Psychogenic Reaction	Diagnosis: Other
In-patients	Mental hospital Unit	11 4% 148 54%	4% 47% } 51%	4% 68% } 72%	72%	55%	70%	54%	50%	33%
Not In-patients	Unit Day- or out-patient General practitioner and other	100 37% 14 5%	45% 4% } 49%	20% 8% } 28%	28%	45%	30%	46%	50%	67%
		273 100%	100%	100%	100%	100%	100%	100%	100%	100%

even the decision between admission to mental hospital or unit seemed influenced by the patient's social class. Comparing the social-class distribution of the mental hospital admissions with that in the sample as a whole, we find if anything there were slightly fewer patients in Classes IV and V amongst the mental hospital admissions than could be expected from the distribution in the total sample; the differences, however, are not significant.

Conclusions

The following general picture emerges from what we found in regard to the events surrounding inception at the units: the psychiatric units were firmly anchored in the medical services; they also provided a varied service, the elderly and physically infirm patients in particular being frequently visited in their homes and coming under psychiatric care without the burden of attendance at an out-patient clinic; and, finally, in the initial stage in-patient admission was freely used, in fact, for the majority of the patients. This usage, however, was selective in the sense that it tended to bring in the elderly, who would find difficulty in frequent attendance as out-patients; it also brought in those who required E.C.T. There seemed to be a slight tendency to treat many schizophrenics on an out-patient basis, although it is true 50% did become in-patients. This particular kind of initial management, which, as we hope to show at a later date, differs from other types of psychiatric care with the same long-term aim, will be tested in what follows against the actual results in the follow-up period and will be shown to be quite important in more than one respect.

Subsequent Care

The main point of interest of our entire investigation was of course to discover whether or to what degree the units had succeeded in their declared policy of avoiding long-term hospitalization, particularly in mental hospital.

We shall here look at the admission of patients to mental hospital first and examine admission as in-patients to the unit separately. Later on we follow this by treating all in-patient admission together.

In order to make the findings presentable in table form and comparable as between the two units, we calculated in each case the sum total of hospital stays over the four years, irrespective of whether the time was spent at one stretch or was composed of a number of short-term stays. This represents what Shepherd (1957) has called the 'total hospital time'. Such a presentation has some disadvantages. There is clearly a fundamental difference between spending three months every year in hospital and staying there for a whole year, yet the two, as presented, will appear indistinguishable. Nevertheless, the method has also some obvious advantages, as it provides a simple figure, which, although not perhaps very descriptive, does give some overall idea of the amount of hospital stay for the whole group of patients in the sample, and illustrates the degree to which they were drawn away from the community.

TABLE 20

Aggregate mental hospital stay over four years

	Time in Mental Hospital			
	None	*Up to 3 Months*	*4–12 Months*	*Over 1 Year*
Blackpool	107 70%	26 17%	6 4%	14 9%
Burnley	113 94%	5 4%	1 1%	1 1%
Both Units	220 81%	31 11%	7 2%	15 6%[1]

[1] Only 0·7% stayed over 2 years.

Mental Hospital Stay

Table 20 shows the 'total hospital time' spent in the mental hospital during the four years of the follow-up period. The most striking finding is that 81% of the total sample never went into mental hospital at all and another 11% only went there for short stays, not exceeding three months in all the four years. A very small number (2%) stayed more than three months, but no longer than one year in all, and only 6% stayed longer than that. Of this 6% (fifteen patients in all), all but two patients stayed less than two years. These two stayed practically the entire period in mental hospital and became truly long-stay patients. This represents a proportion of 0·7%.

Table 20 also shows that there was a difference between the Burnley and Blackpool samples. In the former 94% of the patients never went into mental hospital and another 4% went for less than three months in all. The single patient who stayed longer than a year stayed just less than two years. She was a married woman (thirty to thirty-five years of age) with one child and suffered from schizophrenia. Her illness had already lasted more than two years before inception at the unit, but she had been an active housewife and had also been in employment up to the time she fell ill. Although her condition was already a chronic one when she was first seen at the unit, and in spite of the long duration of her illness, she did spend two of the follow-up years outside hospital. The other longer-stay patient, who was a young man under twenty years of age, also suffered from schizophrenia. He had been living with his parents and had been ill for a considerable time before he came to the unit. He had been a skilled worker previously; his stay in mental hospital in the follow-up period came to just one year. In view of the chronicity of his condition, this was perhaps not unexpected. However, even so, he managed to be fully employed for at least two years out of the three which he spent in the community. At the end of the follow-up period his mental state was assessed as improved. Thus the two people in the Burnley sample who stayed for longish periods in mental hospital were both under sixty years of age and suffered from a chronic type of schizophrenia. But even they spent more than half the follow-up period outside hospital and could be at least in part rehabilitated.

The situation at the Blackpool unit was different. As already indicated, it could not accommodate all those patients who required hospitalization, and had to use the mental hospital beds immediately after inception of the patient. Thus, although only 70% of the patients as compared with 94% in the Burnley sample never went as in-patients in mental hospital, another 17% of the Blackpool patients only stayed there a short time, which is a considerably higher percentage than was the case in Burnley, where there were only 4% of such short-stay patients. The difference probably represents the group of patients who would have stayed in the Blackpool unit if only there had been enough beds. However, we also note here that the longer-stay patients were more numerous in the Blackpool sample as well (4% stayed from four to twelve months as compared with the 1% in the Burnley sample). As many as 7% stayed for one to two years and 2% stayed for more than two years. It should be emphasized once more that these figures represent the 'total hospital time' over the four years and are not necessarily a consecutive hospital stay.

The greater proportion of shorter-stay mental hospital admissions is on the whole adequately explained by the fewer beds at the Blackpool unit. But it is more difficult to explain the larger proportion of long-stay patients entirely in these terms. Shortage of beds may account for some readmissions being channelled into the mental hospital rather than into the unit, but cannot explain why so many patients had a much longer mental hospital experience than in the Burnley sample. Could it be that the very fact that patients have been incepted into mental hospital care exercises a deleterious effect on their later course and makes them more prone to become longer-stay patients than if they had been in-patients in the general hospital units? Certainly these figures seem to suggest that this might be possible.

Neither sex nor age seemed factors which played any important role in bringing the patients into mental hospital. Almost all the patients, particularly the longer-stay ones, were suffering from schizophrenia or an organic psychosyndrome, but the actual numbers were too small for statistical significance. Among the short-term patients, there were a fair number of affective psychoses, probably admitted for purposes of electro-convulsive therapy, but few of these patients spent more than a total of three months through the four years.

Psychiatric Unit Stay

Seeing how little use had been made of mental hospital admissions, even short-stay, as most of them were, the question arises to what extent the patients spent time as in-patients in the psychiatric units.

Table 21 shows that here too most of the admissions were only short-term, and very few patients indeed stayed more than an aggregate of three months throughout the four years. Only 11%

TABLE 21

Aggregate unit in-patient stay

	None		1–4 *Weeks*		5–12 *Weeks*		13 *Weeks and over*[1]	
Blackpool	62	40%	49	32%	29	19%	13	9%
Burnley	31	26%	43	36%	29	24%	17	14%
Both Units	93	34%	92	34%	58	21%	30	11%[1]

[1] 3 patients up to 1 year; 1 patient over 1 year.

fell into this latter category. 34% were never admitted as in-patients at all and another 34% only stayed for less than one month. The majority of them were only in-patients immediately upon inception. With this 68%, therefore, there was no question of long-term stay. Nor was there for the other 21% who during the four years spent no more than three months in the unit. Of the thirty patients (11%) who stayed more than three months, most stayed well under half a year; only three patients stayed longer than that, but no more than one year, and only one patient stayed longer than a year.

As would be expected from the foregoing, there were more patients in the Blackpool sample who never became in-patients in the unit because they were channelled off to mental hospital, as we have indicated, through the shortage of unit beds. As regards the longer-stay patients, there were slightly more in the Burnley unit, where the figure was 14% as compared with 9% in the Blackpool unit. This probably reflects the greater latitude which the larger number of beds allowed the psychiatrist in Burnley. Early discharge was not such a pressing necessity there as with the smaller unit in Blackpool. The differences, however, are not significant.

There were slightly more men than women in the longer-stay group in the Blackpool unit and a slight trend for the older age-group to be admitted and to stay a little longer. Of the diagnostic groups, the schizophrenics were relatively over-represented among the longer-stay patients and to a certain degree the epileptics also. The other diagnostic groups, particularly the affective psychoses, but also the organic psychosyndromes, were under-represented, but none of the above differences was significant. Unlike the mental hospital group, there was a tendency for patients with concomitant non-psychiatric illness, particularly of a chronic type, to spend more time as in-patients in the unit than the patients who were otherwise healthy.

The overall picture then is that, apart from the initial high admission rate, the in-patient facilities of the units were not taxed to any high degree during the four-year follow-up period; in particular, the number of patients staying more than a total of three months was very small indeed, and even the so-called 'longer-stay' patients did hardly ever stay more than one year in all.

TABLE 22

Total in-patient hospital time (unit and mental hospital)

	None		*Up to 3 Months*		*4–12 Months*		*1 Year and Over*	
Blackpool	46	30%	74	48%	20	13%	13	9%
Burnley	30	25%	72	60%	17	14%	1	1%
Both Units	76	27%	146	54%	37	14%	14	5%[1]

[1] 0·7% stayed more than 2 years.

Combined In-patient Stay (Mental Hospital and Unit)

Table 22 shows the combined figures for all in-patient stay, in both the unit and mental hospital. Even when this total in-patient stay is summed up, only 5% are found who spent in all more than one year (25% of the follow-up time) as in-patients in either unit, mental hospital, or both. This is a small proportion indeed. Even if the patients who spent four to twelve months as in-patients are added on, the figure is no higher than 19% of all the patients. In the case of the 27% who spent no time in hospital at all and the 54% who spent under three months (81% in all), there is no question of 'long-term hospital stay'. Of the 5% who stayed more than one year only 0·7% spent more than two years aggregate as in-patients. For all the others (99·3%) the 'total hospital time' was much less than two years, and for 27% of them nil.

The situation in the two units was not very dissimilar, slightly more patients were in-patients of some kind in the Burnley sample, and more were in the short-term category at the unit. This rounds off the impression we formed earlier that the difference between the units here was predominantly due to the fact that the Blackpool unit had too few beds. Not only did this necessitate a larger number of patients having short-term treatment in mental hospital, but the fact that they had to go there seems to have led subsequently to an increase in the number of longer-term patients in that group. Social rehabilitation must start at the moment of inception. The prejudice against mental hospital admission is still very powerful in the public's mind, and hopes for recovery must be lowered when admission to mental hospital takes place; attitudes thus engendered in patients and relatives might well lead to a longer hospital in-patient stay than would in fact be necessary. While we are here trying to explain the differences between the two units, it must not be forgotten that the percentage of patients who stayed in hospital or unit or both for more than 50% of the follow-up time (i.e. more than two years) was a very tiny one indeed (0·7%).

TABLE 23

Total in-patient hospital time
(by age-groups)

	In-patient time			
	None	*Up to 3 Months*	*4–12 Months*	*1 Year and Over*
Age-groups:				
Under-60	33%	47%	15%	5%
Over-60	17%	66%	11%	6%

Table 23 shows that in general the older patient tends to use in-patient facilities more, but this applies only to short stays (under three months); age does not materially affect the longer-stay picture. The diagnostic analysis of the patients shows that the schizophrenics and the organic psychosyndromes were over-represented in the longer-stay group, the schizophrenics were also over-represented in the medium-stay group, while the affective psychoses predominated among the short-term patients. As might be expected, the personality disorders and abnormal psychogenic reactions were more frequent among those patients who never became in-patients at all, but it is noticeable that this latter group also included a number of schizophrenics as well. Table 24 illustrates this point.

TABLE 24

Total hospital in-patient time
(by diagnosis)

	None	*Up to 3 Months*	*4–12 Months*	*1 Year and over*
Organic psychosyndrome and epilepsy	10%	19%	13%	36%
Schizophrenia	17%	19%	43%	43%
Affective psychosis	22%	30%	23%	—
Personality disorder and Abnormal psychogenic reactions	48%	29%	21%	14%
Others	3%	3%	—	7%

Social factors are more often thought to determine length of in-patient stay than are clinical factors, but this did not seem to be the case with our sample, perhaps because relatively few were long-stay in-patients in any case and the small numbers provided rather a slender basis for elaboration of the figures. Table 25 shows that the social-class distribution was not significantly different when patients were separated according to the length of their hospital stay. It will be seen, however, that in the longer-term patients (those staying more than one year) Social Class III was less frequently represented than the others. The difference, however, is not significant.

Civil status also seemed a factor which had but slight influence. The single patients were over-represented in the longer-stay groups, whereas the married patients were over-represented in those who never became in-patients or only for a very short time ($p < 0{\cdot}03$). The widowed, separated, or divorced were more similar to the single patients in this respect.

TABLE 25

Total hospital in-patient time
(by civil status and social class)

Total In-patient Time	*Civil Status*			*Social Class*		
	Single	*Married*	*Widowed, Separated, Divorced*	*I and II*	*III*	*IV and V*
None	25%	65%	10%	17%	50%	33%
Up to 3 months	22%	64%	14%	21%	48%	31%
4–12 months	51%	35%	14%	21%	57%	22%
1 year and over	43%	28%	29%	36%	27%	37%

Conclusions

The main target of the work of these psychiatric units was to avoid long-term hospital stay, and we felt that the figures did indeed show that this aim had been largely achieved in the two units in question. Since the inception of patients into the service was entirely unselective and dealt with all new referrals as they came, this was no mean achievement, and was, we believe, unexpected even by those who organized the services in the first instance (Maclay, 1958). The breakdown of the figures has shown that even where mental hospital admission was arranged and it seemed in very few cases necessary, the majority tended to be quickly discharged. The total group of patients spent by far the greater part of the follow-up period in the community. In the case of the large majority, in-patient admission never occurred, or if it did, this led to a stay of not more than a few weeks over the four years. Well over two-thirds of the patients came into this category.

(*c*) *Effect on the Patient*

Simply to protect the patient from long-term hospital stay seems of course a desirable measure, since we now know that mental illness makes people very vulnerable to such stay, and produces what has been called 'institutionalization'. It, however, cannot be concluded that the management of psychiatric patients extramurally is completely free from any kind of risk. We have examined this group of patients, who, as has been shown, spent very little time in hospital during the four-year follow-up, in order to see if some light could be thrown on this question.

Morbidity and Mortality

Morbidity First of all, it seemed important to know to what extent the patients had actually recovered or otherwise. In order to make our figures comparable we again assessed morbidity in terms of aggregate mental ill-health throughout the four years, i.e. we recorded the total length of time the illness lasted, irrespective of whether this aggregate was made

TABLE 26

Aggregate mental ill-health

		Up to 6 Months	*7–24 Months*	*2 Years and Over*	*Patients*	
					No.	%
Unit	Blackpool	44%	18%	38%	153	100
	Burnley	53%	16%	31%	120	100
	Both units	48%	17%	35%	273	100
Diagnosis	Organic psychosyndrome and epilepsy	31%	25%	44%	42	100
	Schizophrenia	36%	17%	47%	62	100
	Affective psychosis	53%	19%	28%	68	100
	Other	59%	13%	28%	91	100

up of a period of uninterrupted illness or several short spells. Table 26 shows that 48% had been mentally ill for less than six months, 17% had an aggregate duration of mental illness for from seven to twenty-four months, while 35% were ill for more than two years, i.e. for more than 50% of the total time of observation, a considerable number of these in fact for the entire four-year period.

As Table 26 shows, there were slightly more chronically ill patients in the Blackpool unit, but differences were not significant. Over one-third of our total sample, though most of them were out of hospital for the greater part of the time, were by no means well. To this must be added the fact that many of them had a good deal of non-psychiatric disorder. As many as 19% were physically ill for more than two years of the follow-up period; 2–3% were ill for the entire period and another 6% were ill for from seven to twenty-four months. Thus over 25% of the patients had considerable non-psychiatric illness in addition to a good deal of psychiatric morbidity. Many of the non-psychiatric illnesses, moreover, were of a severe kind, some, in fact, terminal illnesses. 17% of the patients died in the course of four years, not counting the 1% who died of suicide. This 17% died of natural causes, cerebral-arteriosclerosis, respiratory disease, etc., and most of them belonged to the upper age-group.

The details of the mortality amongst our group of patients will be discussed in Chapter IV, in particular the question of whether not being in hospital aggravated the mortality rate. It is also feasible to ask whether extramural care might expose patients to more risks of suicide. We will be able to show that this is probably not so.

As regards the psychiatric morbidity, Table 26 also shows, as one would expect, that the different diagnostic groups were affected variously. Personality disorders, abnormal psychogenic reactions and affective psychoses were more numerous among the cases of short-term morbidity (less than one month). It is interesting to know that schizophrenics were by no means absent from that short-term group. As many as 26% fell into this category. This is to be understood in the sense that the florid aspects of the illness passed quickly, leaving only a mild, residual state with few symptoms and not troublesome ones.

In the median range of morbidity, the diagnostic groups were fairly evenly distributed, but in the very chronic group (ill for more than two years) the schizophrenics and the organic psychosyndromes were the most numerous (47% and 44% respectively), but here again personality disorders and abnormal psychogenic reactions were by no means absent; 25% fall into that category.

The age of the patient had a slight effect in that the younger age-group showed slightly more morbidity (50%) than the over-sixty years group (44%), although not to a significant extent.

Employment and Social Adjustment

An objective assessment of the degree of social maladjustment resulting from mental disorder would be a most telling measurement, but it is difficult to come by. One aspect, however, which is relatively easily assessed is the amount of actual unemployment.

A person can during a given period of four years have frequent spells of unemployment or be unemployed for a single long period at a stretch. We have accordingly expressed the total amount of unemployment as a percentage of the total time of the follow-up period, i.e. of the four years. Thus 25% unemployment means a total of one year, 50% means two years unemployment in all, etc.

Unemployment can only be assessed against the expectancy of employment. If someone does not work because he has reached retiring age, it is meaningless to record him as unemployed; we therefore eliminated all patients not of working age as well as the women who had no formal employment and remained as housewives only. There were also a small number of patients on whom no such information could be obtained. This finally left us with a reduced total of 113 patients of working age.

Table 27 shows that of these 113 patients 39% showed no unemployment. In another 16% unemployment was less than 25% of the follow-up time; 37% of the patients, however, were unemployed for more than 50% of the time and 25% of them for more than 75% of the time. This seems a high degree of

TABLE 27

Unemployment during the four years

Amount of Unemployment	*Blackpool*	*Burnley*	*Both Units*	*Men*	*Women*	*Social Class*		
						I and II	*III*	*IV and V*
None	37%	41%	39%	45%	27%	47%	46%	25%
< 25%	13%	22%	16%	11%	27%	24%	13%	17%
25–50%	8%	6%	8%	7%	9%	5%	8%	10%
50–75%	15%	9%	12%	14%	10%	5%	13%	17%
75–100%	27%	22%	25%	23%	27%	19%	20%	31%

unemployment, which in view of the high degree of morbidity is not altogether surprising. In the Blackpool sample there was slightly more unemployment, but the difference was not significant. This might, of course, have been due to factors other than mental illness, such as seasonal trade, etc. As regards long-term unemployment, men and women seemed equally affected, but the men apparently went back to work quicker. Amongst the men 45% had no employment at all, but only 27% of the women. However, if the 'less than one year' unemployment category is added on, the difference between the sexes evens out.

Table 27 also shows that Social Classes IV and V had more unemployment and the figures rise sharply the longer the period of unemployment. These differences are significant ($p < 0{\cdot}05$).

Clinical factors played a part as one would expect. Table 28 shows that there were far more patients suffering from organic psychosyndromes, epilepsy, and schizophrenia in the high unemployment group (40% and 38% respectively), whereas they were relatively less numerous in the fully employed group. Here the other diagnostic groups show a figure of 57%, whereas the organic psychosyndromes and epilepsy are 30% and the schizophrenics only 18%. The dichotomy is not complete. It is remarkable that as many as 18% of the schizophrenics show no unemployment whatsoever, another 23% were unemployed for less than 25% of the time, making a total of 41%, who show relatively little unemployment or none at all through the four years. On the other hand, the other diagnostic groups (consisting mainly of the affective psychoses, personality disorders, and abnormal psychogenic reactions) were not completely absent from the prolonged unemployment group and make their small but definite contribution to it. There were 24% – approximately one-quarter – amongst them who were unemployed for at least 50% of the period or more.

It will, of course, make a difference whether the patient's illness was still fresh when he was incepted or whether he had been ill for a considerable time before. In this latter group one would expect a rather worse social adjustment. This was indeed found to be so. Those patients who had been ill for more than two years before inception showed twice as much long-term

TABLE 28

Unemployment by clinical factors

Proportion of Time Unemployed	*Diagnosis*			*Duration of Illness before Inception*	
	Organic Psychosyndrome and Epilepsy	*Schizophrenia*	*Others*	*Less than 2 Years*	*More than 2 Years*
None	30%	18%	57%	50%	26%
< 25%	10%	23%	13%	17%	17%
25–50%	10%	8%	6%	8%	6%
50–75%	10%	13%	11%	10%	15%
75–100%	40%	38%	13%	15%	36%
	100%	100%	100%	100%	100%

unemployment as those who had been ill for a shorter time.

To complete the above picture of the amount of unemployment in our sample, one must remember the special position of those women who were below retiring age, yet had no formal employment and were *full-time housewives*. The findings here should be seen in conjunction with the previous figures.

In our sample there were only eight such patients, and five out of these eight women were unable to take on any household duties again; they remained unable to do their work for the whole of the four-year period; only one of them showed no 'unemployment' of this kind. The other two women could only manage to look after their homes for something more than two years and were partially disabled for at least 25% of the time. The figures are too small for any further analysis, but the amount of disablement seems larger than among the women who worked outside the home.

As in this unjust world there is no retirement for housewives, we have added the findings on 'unemployment' for the older housewives as well, though we do not know how many women can normally be expected to do full housewives' duties in the upper age-group. Seventy-six older women were described as full-time housewives. Of these more than half coped with their homes for most of the time after inception, but 39% could not cope at all and another 3% coped for less than a year. Although the degree of disablement in this group seems considerable, the proportion of housewives who did return to competence was much higher than with the younger women, where only a minority resumed work at a competent level. It is also fair to say that of those who were counted as unable to cope, a fair proportion continued to do some work with the help of other members of the family or outside social agencies.

Another measure of social maladjustment, less reliable than that of the employment record, is the degree of *social isolation* caused by mental disorder. This is a much more complex situation to assess, and we could only do so rather crudely in the terms of our survey. Social isolation can, of course, have more than one meaning. There is the purely psychological one of 'being lonely', 'feeling solitary'; there is also the purely sociological meaning in the sense of 'absence of social contacts'.

Obviously the two need not coincide. The feeling of loneliness would perhaps be a more sensitive index of the effects of mental disorder, though more difficult to assess in a generally valid way; but it was not possible for us to do more than try to assess social isolation in the second sense, and we did so in terms of the patient's degree of confinement to the home, i.e. was he entirely confined to the house or was he confined most of the time, yet kept a little routine contact (e.g. went to work, shopped nearby his home, etc.) or was he wholly unconfined in his movements? At the end of the four years, we found a considerable degree of confinement: 25·5% were totally confined to the house, 27·5% partially confined. This restriction to the home, even when found among psychiatric patients, need not be attributable to psychiatric illness. We felt, however, that psychiatric illness played some part here in our sample, because at the time of inception only 15·3% of the sample were in no way confined to the home by their illness, but at the time of follow-up this proportion had increased to 47%, while the proportion of those completely confined to the home at inception (60%) had now fallen to 25·5%.

Another finding suggestive of the connection between confinement to the home and psychiatric illness was that the degree of confinement correlated with clinical factors, such as duration of illness and diagnosis, and not so much with the social factors, such as social class, type of household, and so on.

Conclusions

In conclusion, just as there seemed a high degree of morbidity in our sample, there also seemed a fair amount of social maladjustment. The employment situation was not wholly satisfactory, with a considerable amount of prolonged unemployment, and in certain sub-groups, such as the housewives, competence was severely affected. There also seemed reason to believe that social isolation in the sense of impairment of mobility and restriction to the house was also high. The problem which arises is, of course, whether any of this could be avoided and was it due in some way to the extra-mural management? These are important questions, but difficult to answer. Although there did seem a good deal of social maladjustment, some groups of patients where one might expect poor results (e.g. the schizophrenics) did not answer this expectation entirely. A fairly high proportion of them (41 %) were in fact employed for the greater part of the time and did not show any evidence of the confinement to the home.

(*d*) *Effect on Other Services*

The picture gradually emerging now is that although a free use was made of in-patient admissions to the unit, hardly any patients stayed more than a short while and even when re-admitted or, as in a limited number of cases, admission to mental hospital had to be resorted to, the majority of the patients were quickly in and out of hospital. Thus they spent most of the four-year period in the community, with their families, in hostels, lodgings, etc. Yet the patients were by no means well; they had a large amount of persisting mental disorder and on the whole were a physically infirm group, many actually suffering from terminal illness, as shown by the fairly high mortality rate. Had these patients been in mental hospital for this period, the burden of looking after them would have been shouldered by the hospital as part of its routine work. The question arises who in this new extramural service was carrying out the continued care and treatment which many patients needed? One might suspect that demands on other services might increase considerably as a result of shifting the responsibilities of long-term management from in-patients to extramural care. No matter how desirable it may seem to protect such patients from the effects of institutionalization, one may wonder whether other services were adequate to meet the existing needs. We attempted an examination of these circumstances to see whether we could provide some kind of answer.

(*i*) *Other Hospital Psychiatric Services* (*Non-in-patient*)

We first inquired into the demands made by this group of patients on the services provided by the units, other than the in-patient services.

Out-patient Services Since the psychiatrists in charge of the units had their own circumscribed catchment area and had to organize their work in a community-orientated way – that is, not simply provide for patients coming forward for treatment, but feeling a responsibility for a continued service towards the mentally ill members of the community in their catchment area – it was possible that the policy of keeping patients out of hospital beds could only be achieved by frequent supervision through the out-patient department. Patients could, of course, be sent to their out-patients clinic readily by their general practitioners when their illness, for example, created any difficulty at home. We found that a fair number of these patients indeed attended the out-patient clinic, but the numbers did not seem exorbitantly high. We tried to assess this activity quantitatively by counting the number of out-patient attendances, irrespective of whether they fell close together or were scattered widely over the four years. This, of course, represents only a rough estimate of the amount and quality of the out-patient care actually required.

Table 29 shows that 22% of the patients never attended the out-patient department at all during the four-year period. Another 68% attended for less than ten times. The figures include those out-patient attendances that fell into the initial phase after inception. Ten out-patient attendances in four years, keeping the caseload of these units in mind, cannot be construed as demanding anything that could be called intensive work for an out-patient department, even though 68% of the patients required it. Only 10% of the patients had more than ten attendances, and even of these 8% attended no more than twenty-four times and usually much less than that. If the attendances were spread out evenly over the four years, this would amount to one visit every two months, and only 2% attended more than this. Exact figures for comparison elsewhere are lacking, as so far no similar assessment seems to have been made. It does not seem, however, that our figures, such as they are, could represent any excessive burden on an out-patient department. The figures were practically the same for both the units, and there seemed no clinical or social factors that were significant.

Table 29 also shows how the number of out-patient attendances related to the length of time the patient spent as an in-patient, either in the unit or in the mental hospital. If there

TABLE 29

Out-patient attendances by total hospital time

<table>
<tr><th rowspan="2">Total Time in Hospital</th><th colspan="5">Out-patient Attendances</th></tr>
<tr><th>None</th><th>Up to 10</th><th>11–24</th><th>25 and Over</th><th>Total</th></tr>
<tr><td>Less than 3 months</td><td>43 19%</td><td>163 73%</td><td colspan="2">18 8%</td><td>224 100%</td></tr>
<tr><td>4–12 months</td><td>8 23%</td><td>17 50%</td><td colspan="2">9 27%</td><td>34 100%</td></tr>
<tr><td>1 year and over</td><td>10 66%</td><td>5 34%</td><td colspan="2">— —</td><td>15 100%</td></tr>
<tr><td>All patients</td><td>61 22%</td><td>185 68%</td><td>23 8%</td><td>4 2%</td><td>273 100%</td></tr>
</table>

had been a shift of care from the in-patient to the out-patient departments, one would expect to find a large number of attendances in those patients who stayed for a short time in hospital and a smaller number among those who stayed for longer periods. Table 29 does indeed show that such a shift occurs, but only under certain circumstances. The patients who had been in hospital for more than one year seemed to use the out-patient department very little – not one, in fact, attended more than ten times during the four years. But if the hospital time was less than a year, the picture changes. Only 8% of those who spent less than three months in hospital attended as out-patients for more than ten times, but when they had spent from seven months to one year, the figure rises to 27% ($p < 0.05$). The difference is significant and would suggest that the longer-stay group was more ill and therefore required more attention, which was then given partly in the form of more in-patient treatment and partly in the form of more out-patient attendance. One could, of course, speculate whether the in-patient stay could have been further reduced in that group, and what treatment that was necessary could have been given on an out-patient basis, but we are not in a position to answer that question.

As regards the diagnostic groupings, the more frequent attenders suffered in the main from schizophrenia (17%), whereas of the affective psychoses, personality disorders, and abnormal psychogenic reactions the percentage of out-patient attendance was 9–11%. Surprisingly enough, the differences are slight and do not reach statistical significance.

Day-hospital Service Attendances here were rather small. 5% of the patients made use of this service, and only 2% attended the day-hospital for more than a year. It has been pointed out in Chapter II that day-hospital facilities were not yet fully developed at the time of the study. The picture would be different now that the facilities have been extended, at any rate at one of the units. The great use that can be made of such a service has been described in relation to another psychiatric unit not the subject of this study, but also in the Manchester Region (Silverman, 1965).

The number of patients in our sample who attended day-hospital amounted to twenty-six patients, but for some of these the service did represent a great help to themselves and their household and indeed made it possible for them to stay in the community. In this small number had there not been this possibility, long-stay in-patient admission was the likely alternative.

(ii) *General Practitioner Services*

If the expected shift of burden from the in-patient to the out- and day-patient services did not seem to have occurred to any excessive extent, could it be that the patients now living in the community had to be looked after by the family doctor, who then took on the responsibility formerly carried by the hospital?

If the task of assessing out-patient attendance already presents methodological difficulty, the assessment of general practitioner services produces an even greater problem. The method we chose was to count the number of contacts taking place between general practitioner and patient, irrespective of whether they were in the surgery or at home. We realize, of course, that this is barely adequate and can only provide a very crude index indeed. Furthermore, the assessment had to be made in retrospect and relied in many cases on interview-information from patients and relatives and could not be checked. In view of these difficulties, we grouped our findings in broad, descriptive categories, giving the approximate usage of the general-practitioner service within certain defined limits, so as to avoid any misleading pseudo-accuracy. Thus 'infrequent contacts' represented not more than once in six months, 'frequent' represented from two to six consultations in six months, and 'regular' more than once a month.

The high degree of morbidity showed that a change in management can bring all kinds of important changes affecting the patient, but it cannot alter the fact that many psychiatric conditions remain chronic afflictions and take their toll, even though the toll may be reduced owing to the new style of management. If the patient can be spared the dreadful effects of 'institutionalization', this may still seem to be a desirable goal, even though it may not be possible to help him make a completely satisfactory social adjustment by normal standards. We therefore present our findings for what they are worth, with due reservation. As in a number of cases satisfactory information could not be obtained, results are reported on a reduced total of 213 patients.

From our inquiries it appeared that of these 213 patients 11% had no contacts at all through the four-year period, and another 43% had only infrequent ones. A patient seeing his general practitioner twice a year cannot be assessed as an undue burden. Frequent contacts occurred in 13% and regular contacts in 33%. The situation was similar in both units.

TABLE 29A

General practitioner contacts and duration of concomitant physical illness

G.P. Contacts	*Aggregate Duration of Physical Illness*					
	Nil	1–6 *Months*	6–12 *Months*	12–24 *Months*	25 *Months or over*	*Total*
None or infrequent	85%	5%	2%	3%	5%	100%
Frequent or regular	57%	5%	4%	4%	30%	100%

Of course we do not know whether these contacts had been because of a psychiatric complaint or for other types of illnesses. Such an assessment can clearly not be made by retrospective methods; psychiatric illnesses can be brought to the general practitioner, and frequently are, in the disguises of non-psychiatric illness, which may well account for the wide discrepancy in the various assessments of mental disorder in general practice, varying from 2% to 60%. There was, however, a certain amount of indirect evidence in our sample that a number of the general-practitioner contacts were on account of physical illness. Table 29A shows that of the frequent attenders, 30% had physical illnesses lasting more than two years, whereas amongst the infrequent attenders the figure was only 5%. Among the patients with no physical illness or of only short duration, the reverse proportions obtained ($p < 0.001$). The contention that in most cases it was a non-psychiatric complaint that had led to the contact with the general practitioner is also supported by the fact that a significantly higher proportion of frequent and regular attenders fell into the upper age-groups, which are known to have a higher incidence of non-psychiatric illnesses.

Whereas of the under-sixty-year group only 40% had frequent or regular contacts, among the over-sixty-year group the proportion amounted to 66% ($p < 0.001$). Nevertheless, had these patients been in the mental hospital these non-psychiatric conditions should have been attended to there as a matter of course, relieving the general practitioner of this work.

As regards diagnosis, the figures are also shown in Table 30. It was those patients who suffered from affective psychoses and organic psychosyndromes and epilepsy who showed a higher proportion of frequent or regular general-practitioner contacts. The smallest number of frequent or regular contacts appears among the schizophrenics.

If the absolute numbers are taken into consideration, the burden on the general practitioner created by these patients does not seem excessively large. Since our figures could not be based on exact records and represent only an approximate estimate, their interpretation cannot be pressed too far. However, comparing them with due reservation, with those given by Logan and Cushion (1958) for the general population, our sample of patients contacted their general practitioners on the average twice as often as the national average – namely, they had 12·3 contacts on average per annum as compared with six per annum as the national average.

Of course, a group of patients all of whom had initially been referred to a hospital must be expected to require more medical services in the subsequent years, including the general-practitioner services, than would be the case with the average population. Our comparison, therefore, might be thought unwarranted. What one would like to know is how many contacts would the general practitioner have had to deal with in a similar group of patients all of whom had a mental disorder severe enough at one stage to lead to referral to a hospital? How many contacts would he have had to deal with had these

TABLE 30

General practitioner contacts

General Practitioner Attendances	*Patients*		*Age-groups*		*Diagnoses*			
			Under 60	*Over 60*	*Organic Psychosyndrome and Epilepsy*	*Schizophrenia*	*Affective Psychosis*	*Others*
None	23	11%	60%	34%	46%	74%	38%	62%
Infrequent	92	43%						
Frequent	28	13%	40%	66%	54%	26%	62%	38%
Regular	70	33%						

patients been under more conventional methods of management, allowing for more in-patient care? As yet no such figures appear to exist.

Re-referrals Perhaps another index of the involvement of the general practitioner is the number of times he has to re-refer his patient formally to the unit. This occurred in 28% of our sample, but only in 8% was there need for more than one such re-referral in the four-year period. This is not a negligible figure perhaps, and it reflects to a certain extent the degree of co-operation that existed between the units and the general-practitioner service. The figures were similar in the two units, and this interplay between the units on one hand, which discharge patients early and only keep a limited number on as out-patients, and the general practitioner, on the other, who readily re-refers patients discharged but now requiring further hospital attention, is the expected pattern of an extramural service.

Domiciliary Visits Equally, the number of domiciliary visits which took place during the follow-up period could also be seen as an index of this co-operation between unit and general practitioner. Here, however, we found that, while the number of re-referrals appeared fairly large, the number of domiciliary visits paid during the follow-up period was very small – namely, 4% as opposed to the rather high figure (25%) of patients who had had domiciliary visits on inception. At inception the older age-group had received more visits than the under-sixty-year age-group, but this age difference was not apparent among those who received subsequent visits. This may be partly due to the fact that the over-sixty-year age-group tended to diminish through the four years owing to deaths. In any case, absolute numbers were small and it would be difficult to carry interpretation beyond a certain point. No single diagnostic group predominated, except that no domiciliary visits were paid to patients with personality disorders or abnormal psychogenic reactions.

Social-class distinctions were not very marked in respect to the visits at inception, but were distinctly more so in the subsequent visits, where Social Classes I and II were more highly

TABLE 31

Domiciliary visits

		None		*At Inception Only*		*During the Follow-up Period*		*All Patients*	
Social Class	I & II	38	68%	11	20%	7	12%	56	100%
	III	82	67%	40	32%	2	1%	124	100%
	IV & V	61	79%	14	18%	2	3%	77	100%
Age-groups	Under 60 years	148	80%	30	16%	6	4%	184	100%
	Over 60 years	44	50%	39	44%	6	6%	89	100%
All patients		192	71%	69	25%	12	4%	273	100%

represented than the rest – in fact, three times as high. This difference is highly significant ($p < 0{\cdot}001$). This would suggest that whereas in the initial referral the decision to ask for a domiciliary visit was guided by clinical factors, with subsequent visits the decision was to a certain extent prompted by the social-class status of the patient.

(*iii*) *General Hospital Services*

Kidd (1962 *a* and *b*) has shown that psychiatric patients, particularly in the older age-groups, are often admitted to general wards. This type of misplacement, which, as Kidd indicated, may have serious consequences, can arise with considerable frequency even where there is a mental hospital service in easy reach for long-term hospitalization. We had to exclude that such admissions to general hospital were in fact taking place in our own group of patients. There were indeed a number of general hospital admissions during the four-year period – namely, 23% – but 20% represented stays of less than three months. All these patients had non-psychiatric illnesses, but it may nevertheless have been that the fact of their psychiatric illness was a contributing factor to their admission to general hospital. This possibility cannot be eliminated, but since the total hospital time spent by the 20% was less than three months over the four years, this cannot be regarded as 'prolonged hospitalization' and as any substitute for 'prolonged mental hospital stay'. The fact that they stayed only a short period is highly suggestive that the main cause for admission was non-psychiatric illness and that there was no 'misplacement' in Kidd's sense of the term. Most were in the older age-groups, though not all: only 3% of the group stayed longer than three months. As far as we could ascertain, they all in fact suffered from serious physical illnesses (tuberculosis, diabetes, etc.), which in their own right warranted hospital admission.

(*iv*) *Social Services*

The National Health Service Act, 1946, established the division of responsibilities between the hospital and the local authority, placing the social care of patients living in the

TABLE 32A

Amount of social agency care

Social Agency (Statutory)	Number of Patients receiving Help Total Number, 230		
	None	*Occasional*	*Frequent*
Mental Health Service	69%	28%	3%
Health visitors	98%	1%	1%
Home help	96%	1%	3%
District nurses	94%	4%	2%
Social Welfare	99%	1%	—
Housing Department	100%	—	—
National Assistance Board	88%	4%	8%
Ministry of Pensions and National Insurance	99%	1%	—
Ministry of Labour	90%	12%	—
Children's Department	99%	1%	—
Probation Service	99%	1%	—
Any other agency	95%	3%	2%

community on the shoulders of the latter. In the case of the conventional mental hospital service, this usually meant in-patients who had been discharged from hospital. But with the group of patients under survey local authority responsibility began much earlier, often without the patient entering hospital at all. Although the division of responsibility between the two authorities has its own justification, it has at an early stage been pointed out that unless the two services are closely integrated the care may become discontinuous and the patient suffer. It has been advocated that the National Health Service psychiatric adviser, usually in the person of the hospital superintendent, should become the psychiatric adviser to the Medical Officer of Health (Macmillan, 1956). In the catchment areas of the two units studied this co-ordination has been largely realized. The psychiatrist in charge of the unit was in fact adviser to the Medical Officer of Health and the two public services run hand in hand, with the mental welfare officers working directly with the unit psychiatrist.

We examined the contribution of the services rendered to our group of patients by the local authority mental health department, but we also cast our net wider to include other statutory social services not directly under the Medical Officer of Health, as well as voluntary agencies.

Tables 32A and 32B list all the statutory and voluntary agencies used and records the number of patients who received help from each. It can be seen that the help given by most agencies was marginal over the four years. The most extensive contribution was made, as might be expected, by the mental health service (28% of the sample received occasional help, but only in a further 3% was such help frequent). 12% received occasional help from the Ministry of Labour. The National Assistance Board also made some contribution (4% of the sample received occasional help, 8% frequent help). The District Nurse gave occasional help to 4% and frequent help to 2%, while the Home Help service gave 1% occasional help and 3% frequent help. These last two agencies were mostly concerned with the old age-group. The remaining agencies in general gave help to only 1% or 2% of the patients at most. Thus the total amount of help given by the statutory agencies cannot be considered very large over the four years. 2% of the patients received help from voluntary sources. Where patients were employees (11%), this sort of help came mostly, in nearly two-thirds of such cases, from employers themselves: 8% were

TABLE 32B

Amount of social agency care

Social Agency (Voluntary)	*Number of Patients receiving Help Total Number, 230*		
	None	*Occasional*	*Frequent*
Voluntary organizations	98%	1%	1%
Church or chapel	99%	1%	—
Help at Work:	89%	11%	—
from employer		64%	
from Personnel Dept.		8%	
from foreman		12%	
from colleagues		16%	

helped by the personnel department; less formal help was given by foreman or departmental heads in 12% or by colleagues at work (16%). Two individuals were helped by their church or chapel.

In several cases, of course, there was an overlap of services, and one patient would receive help from a number of sources. The total picture indicating the amount of help received, irrespective of source is shown in Table 33.

TABLE 33

Amount of social agency care
(by units and social class)

	Number of Patients who received Social Agency Care			
	None	*Occasional*	*Periodic*	*Constant*
Blackpool	60%	25%	6%	9%
Burnley ...	50%	37%	7%	6%
Both units	55%	30%	7%	8%
Social Class I & II	66%	23%	2%	9%
Social Class III	79%	44%	6%	7%
Social Class IV & V	44%	31%	15%	10%

With forty patients this question did not apply or no reliable answer could be elicited; this left a total of 233 patients. Of these 85% received no social help or only of a very occasional nature. In 7% help was offered periodically and in 8% the social help was almost constant. The figures appeared much the same in both units, although the patients at the Burnley unit received slightly more occasional help. The differences are not significant.

The help received was the same for those aged under sixty and over sixty years, but the older people had more constant help, while with the younger group periodic help was the more frequent. This was probably related to the higher morbidity rate among the elderly. There was no relationship to the diagnostic grouping, except that with the schizophrenics periodic social help was the more common. Figures are small, however, and too much cannot be made of the differences.

Table 33 shows that there is a slight gradient related to social status in that the Social Classes I and II received the least periodic or constant social care (11%); the figures for Class III were 13% and for Classes IV and V 25% ($p < 0.005$). Also, slightly more single persons (15%) received social help than the married (14%), but the difference is not significant.

Thus clinical factors seemed to be of less significance than the social factors, which is not unexpected. The fact that so relatively little help was offered does not mean, of course, that more might not have been done. We could not assess the objective need for social-agency help and there were no figures available to provide any basis for comparison. We did, however, ask the large proportion of patients (85%) who had received no social help over the four years, or only very occasionally, why this was so. We found that 89% of them said they had felt no need. In the other 11% help would have been appreciated, but 8% had been reluctant to ask. For the rest, either the patient or the relatives had not known how to go about it or did not know what help was available.

The above figure (11%) is small, but gives some indication that the social services in these catchment areas did not reach all who could have benefited from their efforts.

(*e*) *The Burden of the Family*

From the point of view of the psychiatric administrator, the picture that has emerged so far is an encouraging one. A completely unselected group of psychiatric patients has been managed over a period of four years in such a way that they were kept out of long-stay mental hospital beds and spent most of their time in the community. The relief of the in-patient services was not achieved at the expense of other branches, such as the out-patient, day-patient, or domiciliary services, nor at the expense of the general hospital service, nor yet of the general practitioner. All these other services may have taken a greater share in looking after these patients than would have been the case if these latter had spent most of their time in mental hospital, but the figures show that this increase was not of any magnitude, and none of these services could be described as overloaded with the care of such patients.

Yet the patients themselves were by no means all recovered, there was a good deal of mental and physical morbidity among them, and their social adjustment was by no means complete. Many did not return to become breadwinners or look after their homes and children, and many during their continued illness or relapse displayed abnormal behaviour and withdrawal which must have been a source of distress to those around them.

Critics of this type of extramural care may well ask whether the burden of care was not merely shifted on to the patients' families. Wing *et al.* (1964*b*) indeed, in following up a group of mental hospital patients discharged to their homes, found that in many instances the patients could only stay there if the families were prepared to act as 'nurses'. This is clearly a problem which cannot be ignored, and as more and more psychiatric work orientates itself towards keeping patients in the community more attention has to be directed to this aspect.

The investigation of such family burden, however, is relatively new and methods of assessment have still to be developed. We have tried to assess the burden on the families of the patients in our sample, and will set out the particular methods we employed.

Method of Assessment

Our main problem was how to assess the ways in which the patients affected their households and the extent to which they in fact did so. Grad and Sainsbury (1963) were pioneers in this field, having become aware of the problem in relation to a mental hospital service, which was directed towards the same aims as the general hospital psychiatric units – namely, that of keeping the patients out of hospital as much as possible. They evolved certain methods which seemed to offer an approach whereby one could tackle this problem, and with their co-operation we made the fullest use of these, adapting them to our own purpose of investigating two general hospital psychiatric units by means of a four-year follow-up study.

Grad and Sainsbury's methods were geared to an established institution and a different type of service; they were used for a progressive investigation and, since ours was a retrospective study, some alterations had to be made. Nevertheless, where changes were necessary, they were done in such a way as to keep findings as comparable as possible.

Grad and Sainsbury (1963) used the word 'burden' to describe and summarize certain adverse effects on the family created by the patient's illness, and we have adopted the expression. It does, however, require some care in its usage, because the investigated and the investigator may have different conceptions on the matter. It is of very great importance to particularize and define clearly which areas of stress are being inquired into. Our own definition can be presented as follows:

The areas of inquiry respecting 'burden' fall into the two following large groups, the individual items of which are largely in line with those tabulated by Grad and Sainsbury:

(1) Certain specific effects on the daily life of the household.
(2) The occurrence of certain abnormal behaviour in the patient, with the assumption that such occurrence (if periodic or constant) must by itself represent some burden on the household.

These two different groups each constitute what we have called the 'objective' burden on the household. When the two are put together, we have used the term 'combined objective burden'.

We also inquired whether the household members themselves had felt that they were carrying a burden during the four years. This we called the 'subjective' burden.

It will be seen that in the event 'objective' and 'subjective' burdens by no means coincided. In fact, having made this distinction, it was not only possible to relate the two types of burden to each other, but to a number of clinical and social factors as seemed relevant.

'Objective' Burden

Table 34 lists the varied adverse effects on the household due to the patient's illness. They have been grouped under four headings, (1) financial, (2) health, (3) effects on children,

TABLE 34

'Objective' burden
(Adverse effects on the household)

Type of 'Objective' Burden caused by Patient's Illness		*Percentage of Households affected*
Financial	Financial status of the patient or of the household has suffered	16·5%
	Any member of the household lost earnings	6·6%
	Any member of the household had to start going out to work	5·1%
Health	Physical strain on any member of the household, due to nursing the patient	some, 4·4% marked, 1·5%
	Poor health in any member of the household, caused by patient's illness	6·9%
Children	Separation of children under 16	from mother, 7·3% from father, 5·1% from both, 0·4%
	Distress in children under 16	distressed, 2·1% neurotic, 0·4%
General	Disruption of the life of any member of the household	some, 25·7% marked, 12·8%

(4) effects on family routine, e.g. interruption of social life, of children's schooling, etc. The highest percentage of households were affected under the fourth heading (38·5%). If, however, only severe effects are taken into account, the figure drops to 12·8%. Next in frequency came financial loss to the patient (16·5%), loss of earnings to other members of the household (6·6%), while in 5% other family members were forced to go out to work as a direct result of the patient's illness.

General physical strain on others occurred in 5·9%, but if severe cases only are counted, the figure was no more than 1·5%. In 6·9% there was an actual breakdown into illness. Separation of children from their parents occurred in 12·8% of the cases. This is not an inconsiderable figure, and in 2·5% the child seemed disturbed or frankly neurotic as a result. It should be remembered, however, that this item only applied to families where there were young children present, which meant about 25% of the sample.

If we take only these families at risk, then 40·7% underwent separation, by which is meant separation lasting longer than a week, and the figure for distress in the children then amounts to 8·1%.

TABLE 35

'Objective' burden
(abnormal behaviour)

Types of Abnormal Behaviour	*Constant*	*Periodic*	*Occasional*
Noisy or wandering at night	3·6	4·7	1·1
Dangerous to themselves or others	4·7	7·7	4·7
Unacceptable sexual behaviour	0·7	0·7	—
Generally restless, noisy or talkative	0·7	7·3	21·2
Unresponsive	2·5	4·1	1·5
Apparently wilfully unco-operative	5·1	10	2·1
Used odd speech or expressed 'unusual ideas'	4·4	11·3	3·3
Hypochondriasis	4·4	0·7	0·7
Requiring physical or nursing care	10·6	4·4	2·7
Demanding excessive companionship	5·5	3·3	2·1
Other unusual behaviour	10·9	14·6	3·3

Table 35 lists the other aspect of 'objective' burden, that of patients' abnormal behaviour. We recorded the degree of its occurrence, i.e. whether constant, periodic, or occasional during the four-year period. We assumed that when any such behaviour occurred more than occasionally it must constitute some form of burden to those around the patient.

Most types of abnormal behaviour showed a fairly low incidence of burden, affecting some 10% of the patients (if we take constant and periodic occurrence together). Behaviour that occurred more widely than this was as follows: that broadly grouped under the heading 'other unusual behaviour' (25·5%).

This included (1) hostile, irritable, morose behaviour, (2) behaviour calling for supervision or watchfulness, e.g. the forgetfulness of dementia, (3) offensive personal habits, (4) extreme seclusiveness and withdrawal. Three other items, 'unco-operative behaviour', 'odd speech and unusual ideas' (in deluded patients), and 'the need for nursing care' also occurred with somewhat greater frequency (approximately 15% in each case). Thus although the majority of patients did not seem to have displayed abnormal behaviour, a fair proportion did so either periodically or constantly in the four years, which cannot have failed to cause some stress in their environment.

No account is taken in Table 35 as to whether only one or several of the respective stresses coincided in one and the same household, but, of course, a certain amount of overlap did occur.

The similarities and differences of these two types of 'objective' burden in relation to other clinical and social factors have been analysed in more detail elsewhere (Hoenig and Hamilton, 1966), and although we found certain divergencies, it still seemed justifiable and illuminating for purposes of comparison to put them together into a single total. We accordingly drew into one group all households where *any* 'objective' burden had occurred, irrespective of the specific type to which it belonged. Thus emerged what we called the 'combined objective burden', which represented the sum total of all the types of burden listed severally above.

We found that there were 152 patients (55·7%) where some 'objective' burden had been recorded, as against 121 patients (44·3%) where no 'objective' burden appeared, or where, in the case of abnormal behaviour, this had occurred only occasionally in the four-year time. Having established this, it seemed important to see what other factors related to the 'combined objective burden' in this general sense.

Such factors as sex, age, civil status, and social class seemed unrelated to the incidence of this burden. But whether the patient lived with parents, spouse, or in some other setting did seem to make some difference.

Table 36 shows that patients living with their parents formed only 18·4% of the 'burden' group, as compared with 28·1% of the 'no burden' group ($p < 0·05$). Patients who lived with their

TABLE 36

'Combined objective' burden
(by type of household)

Type of Patient's Home	*With Parents*	*With Spouse*	*With Other Kin*	*Living Alone or Without Fixed Abode*	*Total*
No 'burden'	28·1%	38·8%	11·5%	21·6%	100%
'Burden'	18·4%	59·2%	13·9%	8·5%	100%

spouses showed a reverse trend (59·2%) in the 'burden' group compared with 38·8% in the 'no burden' group (p. $<0·01$). Those living with other kin are equally represented in both groups. Thus the parental home appeared to suffer less than the conjugal home. Those who lived alone or with no fixed abode were relatively more prominent in the 'no burden' group, no doubt due to the absence of any household of their own to carry the burden during the four years. The implications of the differences between the parental and conjugal homes will be discussed later.

As regards clinical factors, the expected differences do not appear between the 'burden' and 'no burden' groups. The diagnostic groupings are fairly equally represented in both, and the small differences that occur are not significant. The morbidity rate, on the other hand, seemed more significant. Patients who were ill for more than two years of the follow-up period comprised 65·2% of the 'burden' group as compared with 23% of the 'no burden' group ($p<0·001$). There is a consistent decrease in the 'burden' group, the shorter the duration of the illness. In the 'no burden' group the trend goes consistently in the other direction ($p<0·001$). The differences shown in Table 37 are very highly significant. The longer the

TABLE 37

'Combined objective' burden
(by morbidity)

Aggregate Duration of Illness during 4 Years	*Up to 6 Months*	*7–24 Months*	*25 Months and over*	*Total*
No burden	45·9%	31·1%	23%	100%
Burden	10·8%	24%	65·2%	100%

patients were ill, the more likely they were to cause some 'objective' burden to their household. The quickly recoverable conditions caused least upset, independently of the diagnostic categories. The total hospital time, i.e. the aggregate time spent as an in-patient over the four years, also seemed related to the 'objective' burden. It will be remembered that the total hospital time spent as in-patient was assessed through the four

TABLE 38

'Combined objective' burden
(by total hospital time)

Total Hospital Time	*Nil*	*Up to 3 Months*	*4–12 Months*	*1 Year and Over*	*Total*
No burden	42%	28%	22·3%	7·7%	100%
Burden	16·4%	26·3%	30·9%	26·4%	100%

years, whether the stay was consecutive or intermittent, as indeed it was for the large majority. Those who had been in-patients for more than one year composed 26·4% of the 'burden' group, as against 7·7% of the 'no burden' group. The figures in the medium-stay group show the same type of difference, if less well marked. Those patients, however, who did not enter hospital at all constituted 16·4% of the 'burden' group and 42% of the 'no burden' group ($p < 0·001$). It is not easy to interpret these figures. If one assumes that increasing burden leads to more hospitalization, one would expect the aggregate hospital stay to lengthen accordingly. On the other hand, could it be that hospitalization might actually be the cause of the 'burden' – involving financial loss, separation of children, etc.? Without being able to settle this, we suspect that the length of hospital stay was a result of burden rather than a producer of it.

It is impossible to say whether the absolute incidence (55%) of this 'combined objective burden' was unduly large in our group of patients. In actual figures it seems considerable, affecting more than half of the households. The fact that it was sensitive to such factors as type of household, duration of illness, and possibly total hospital stay suggests it has some validity as a measure of household burden where psychiatric illness occurs.

'Subjective' Burden

Independently of the inquiry relating to 'objective' burden, the informants other than the patient, wherever available, were asked whether as a result of the patient's illness they themselves thought the household had suffered a sense of burden over the four years. This was an inquiry not so much into the 'objective' facts as into attitudes. It was striking to find that these 'subjective' attitudes by no means corresponded with what one might have expected from the assessment of the 'objective' burden.

The figures for 'subjective' burden could only apply to those informants who were associated with the patient for the whole four-year period. This finally reduced our total to 179 cases. Of these we found that 45·8% reported no 'subjective' burden, 40·2% reported a moderate degree, and 13·9% a severe degree of burden. Tables 39–42 refer to this 'subjective' burden as related to the combined 'objective' burden.

TABLE 39

'Subjective' burden
(by 'combined objective' burden)

'Subjective' Burden	*'Combined Objective' Burden*	
	No Burden	*Burden*
None	100%	23·6%
Some burden	—	56·7%
Severe burden	—	19·6%
All patients	—	100%

Table 39 shows that where no combined 'objective' burden had been recorded, there was, as one might expect, no 'subjective' burden. It should be remembered that in a number of these cases, very occasional 'objective' burden had arisen (which for our purpose we had counted as 'no burden' over the four years), but this occasional burden had obviously been accepted by the families and within the conspectus of the four-year period was not seen as any matter of complaint.

Where, however, more than occasional 'objective' burden had arisen, informants complained about severe 'subjective' burden in 19·6% of the cases; another 56·7% had complained of some 'subjective' burden. Thus in 76·3% of the households where the patient had caused 'objective' burden of some kind, this had been experienced as a 'subjective' burden by the family. The most interesting group perhaps were those households where 'objective' burden had arisen, but it had not been experienced as any hardship at all, nor was any complaint expressed (23·6%). This was nearly a quarter of all the families with some 'objective' burden. This figure might therefore be regarded as a kind of measure of the family tolerance towards the psychiatric patient.

'Subjective' burden seemed on the whole more sensitive to the various factors examined than the combined 'objective' burden; for instance, the age factor seemed to play a part. Although both the under-sixty and the over-sixty age-group did not differ in the amount of 'objective' burden carried by their households, there was significantly more 'subjective' burden in the households of the older age-group (50·5% of the households of the under-sixty age-group were in the 'no burden' category, compared with only 36·5% of the over-sixty age-group, $p < 0 \cdot 05$). The difference is maintained if only severe 'subjective' burden is compared (21·6% of the over-sixty age-group created 'severe' burden compared with 10% of the under-sixty age-group).

Severe 'subjective' burden was also greater where there were married patients, who comprised 76% of this category, whereas single patients (including the widowed, divorced and separated) constituted only 24% ($p < 0 \cdot 001$). This might well have been related to the fact that the conjugal homes had a larger amount of 'objective' burden to carry.

Table 40 shows that the type of household had some effect on the situation. Where patients lived with siblings or other kin, 'subjective' complaint was least (in 41·3%). Where they lived with their spouses the figure was 50%, and where they lived with their parents 60·4%. The highest figure (80%) occurred where patients lived with their grown-up children ($p < 0 \cdot 02$). There is a discrepancy here from what was found in relation to the combined 'objective' burden (Table 36). Outstanding is the parental home, which, although it appeared to suffer less 'objective' burden, has one of the highest 'subjective' burden rates. This would suggest that the parental home is more intolerant and reacts more severely to the sick person than do the other types of household.

TABLE 40

'Subjective' burden

'Subjective' Burden	*Living with Parents*	*Living with Spouse*	*Living with Grown-up Children*	*Living with Other Kin*	*Living Alone or of No Fixed Abode*
None	39·6%	49·5%	20%	58·7%	50%
Some burden	52·6%	33·7%	60%	35·3%	37%
Severe burden	7·8%	16·3%	20%	6%	13%
All patients	100%	100%	100%	100%	100%

Whereas 'objective' burden showed no relationship to social class, the 'subjective' burden appeared greater in Social Classes I (66·6%) and II (62%), whereas the figures for Classes III, IV and V respectively were 49·4%, 47%, and 48%. If severe 'subjective' burden is taken alone, the trend is similar (24% in Class II, 16·8% in Class III, 6% and 9% in Classes IV and V). The trends are consistent, but the differences are not statistically significant.

There were some differences in the diagnostic groupings, but they did not reach statistical significance either. The families of epileptics (75%), organic psychosyndromes (70%), and schizophrenics (69·4%) showed the highest incidence of 'subjective' burden. Those of patients with personality disorders (43%) or abnormal psychogenic reactions (41·3%) showed the lowest. Families of those patients suffering from organic psychosyndromes were also associated with the highest incidence of *severe* 'subjective' burden. It is interesting to note that the schizophrenics caused little severe burden as compared with the organic psychosyndromes and affective psychoses. Since it has been shown that 'objective' burden for the households of the schizophrenics was as high as with the other diagnostic groups, there would seem to be a particular form of tolerance towards them. Relatively few gave rise to any severe complaints in their households and the majority of complaints seemed to be of a mild nature.

TABLE 41

'Subjective' burden
(by aggregate morbidity)

'Subjective' Burden	*Duration of Illness during the 4 Years*			
	Up to 6 Months	*7–12 Months*	*13–24 Months*	*25 Months and Over*
None	67%	45%	12·5%	21·1%
Some burden	33%	35%	81·5%	50·5%
Severe burden	—	20%	6%	28·1%
Total	100%	100%	100%	100%

Table 41 shows the relationship between 'subjective' burden and the aggregate morbidity. The least 'burden' appears related to those patients who had been ill for less than six months (33%, $p < 0.001$) and those ill from seven to twelve months (55%). The figure then rises steeply for those ill for from one to two years (87·5%, $p < 0.05$). Once, however, the two-year period is over, the figure is seen to fall slightly to 78·6%, suggesting that some adjustment might have been made by the household concerned.

As regards severe 'subjective' burden, however, apart from the fact that none arose among the households of those patients ill for less than six months, the general trend was not maintained as clearly, since, when morbidity lasted from seven to twelve months, a considerable amount of severe complaint arose (20% as compared with 6% in the one-to-two-year group).

TABLE 42

'Subjective' burden
(by total hospital time)

'Subjective' Burden	*Total Hospital Time during 4 Years, in Weeks*				
	None	*Up to 4*	5–12	13–52	53 *and over*
None	62%	55%	41·5%	21·8%	10%
Some burden	31%	35·3%	32%	74%	70%
Severe burden	7%	9·7%	26·5%	4·2%	20%
All patients	100%	100%	100%	100%	100%

The relationship between 'subjective' burden and the 'total hospital time' spent by patients as in-patients shows similar trends, as can be seen in Table 42. Those patients who had never been in hospital created 'subjective' burden in 38% of the cases, those whose stay only totalled up to four weeks in 45% of the cases, while those whose stay totalled from five to twelve weeks created complaints in 58·5%. There is a steep rise to 78·2% for those who stayed from three months up to one year and to 90% for those over one year ($p < 0.01$). The differences are not quite so marked if severe 'subjective' burden is considered alone, the highest percentage appearing in the five-to-twelve-week group (25·6%).

Both as regards the 'total hospital time' and the 'aggregate morbidity', one notes a levelling of effect in relation to the 'subjective' burden after the second year in each case. This is unlike what was found in relation to 'objective' burden, and seems to imply that the households make some adjustment to the illness and after that length of time a degree of tolerance develops.

Conclusions

For the evaluation of our findings we have to depend only on intra-group comparison. Figures are not yet available that would allow comparison with groups of patients who have been differently managed or treated. From internal comparison we can see that the fairly large 'objective' burden was in many cases accepted without complaint and that there was a good deal of tolerance extended toward psychiatric patients in their homes. The severe 'subjective' burden was in fact not as high as might have been expected. It seemed linked with certain diagnostic groups and with the duration of the patient's illness. There seemed no doubt that some suffering in the households had been caused over the four years by the patient's particular psychiatric illness, but whether any of this was due to the specific type of management is difficult to assess. Perhaps more light can be thrown on this important question in the following section, when we come to examine the attitudes of patients and relatives to various aspects of the service.

(*f*) *Consumer attitudes*

Doctors and medical administrators tend to assume that what they believe to be right for the patient and in his best interests will also be seen in this same light by the patient and his relatives. However, the new administrative arrangement under review in this survey, which to the doctors seems a measure of protection for the patient against institutionalization, may appear to question this assumption. Indeed, one of the most striking characteristics – the policy of keeping patients out of mental hospital and in the community as much as possible – could be seen by the relatives as withdrawal of shelter for the chronic patient and a shift of some of the burden of caring for him on to his household. From the doctors' and administrators' point of view, the intention, of course, is to keep the patient in an environment which will be less damaging to him than that of an institution, however well run, and from what we have shown so far there seems good ground for this view, and the new administrative arrangements may be said to work. But was all this seen in the same light by the patients and their relatives? This seemed to us a not unimportant question to ask, and we examined the answers in some detail.

In doing so, we were not, of course, dealing with objectively ascertainable facts, but with elicited attitudes. We were carrying out what may be called an 'opinion poll'. Such a procedure is always fraught with danger if conclusions are drawn too hastily. The answers to our questions were given by people who were personally deeply involved in the situation, and this was bound to have emotional repercussions. Furthermore, in the case of the patients there was the additional difficulty that many of them were not quite recovered or well at the time of the interview.

We tried to keep all this clearly in mind when we analysed the findings. It should be emphasized that the questions were not put in a completely structured way to the patients and relatives, but formed part of a long and searching interview during which the research worker aimed to create an atmosphere of trust, so that the probands could be given the best opportunity for a frank expression of opinion. Furthermore, whatever the opinion given, the proband's intention could also be explored at the time by the research worker. We are aware that this procedure has weaknesses, but the method, if carefully applied, is perhaps not quite as unreliable as one might fear.

Tolerance towards the Patient

Household attitudes are likely to be influenced by what the family members feel about psychiatric illness as such. This *in abstracto* is difficult to elicit in any way that would yield valid answers. We asked a variety of questions directed to finding out what the informants felt was the matter with the patient, what was the attitude to mental illness as such, did they prefer to call it by some other name, etc.? But the answers obtained led us to abandon any attempt to evaluate them. We also directed a question at the family's attitude to the particular illness with which they were faced, what they felt about the patient's illness at the time of inception, and we classified the answers according to whether they were sympathetic or unsympathetic. Only 10% of the informants gave answers which could be classified as unsympathetic, involving such answers as being afraid of the patient, feeling it was his fault, that he was not really ill, had become a nuisance, etc. Factors which might have brought on such a rejecting attitude were examined, but such differences as were found did not reach statistical significance. The age of the patient, for instance, did not matter. Diagnoses of personality disorder and epilepsy were over-represented in the 'unsympathetic' category, organic psycho-syndromes and affective psychoses were equally represented, while the diagnosis most over-represented in the 'sympathetic' group proved to be that of schizophrenia. There was also some correlation with the length of time the patient spent in hospital over the four years, but this could have been the source of 'unsympathetic' attitudes rather than their consequence. The longer the aggregate hospital stay, the more likely it was that the patient was met with unsympathetic attitudes in the home. Different lengths of stay were looked at separately, and the above trend seemed constant throughout, but the differences did not reach statistical significance.

At the end of the four years attitudes had not changed very much from those at inception. The percentage of those who did not enjoy sympathetic support from the other family members was 8%. There were similar relationships with age of patient and aggregate hospital time as at inception. The clinical outcome did seem to correlate to some extent with the sympathy extended to the patient, since the worse the outcome of his illness the less he enjoyed any sympathy.

On the whole, therefore, our patients seem to have had a considerable measure of sympathetic support, both at inception and during the subsequent four years of extramural care. Attitudes did not change very much, with unsympathetic attitudes reducing slightly, but remaining about the 10% level.

TABLE 43

Informant's attitude to patient's illness at time of inception (by diagnosis)

Informant's Attitude to the Illness	*All Cases*		*Diagnostic Categories*					
			Organic Psychosyndrome	*Schizophrenia*	*Affective Psychosis*	*Epilepsy*	*Personality Disorder Abnormal Psychogenic Reactions*	*Others*
Sympathetic	143	90%	19%	24%	26%	2%	27%	2%
Not sympathetic	15	10%	13%	13%	20%	7%	40%	7%

It would be interesting to know whether this small percentage of antagonistic feelings to psychiatric distress is characteristic of other areas or not, but we know of no suitable comparison.

Within this general context of sympathetic response to the patient's illness, we come to consider one of the attitudes which has already been touched upon in an earlier section, what we have called the sense of 'subjective' burden. We have seen that this by no means coincided with the actual 'objective' burden which can be recorded in fact for the family. There were nearly a quarter of the households (23·6%) where, although 'objective' burden indubitably existed, the household members had not experienced it as any burden. If one restricts oneself to the sense of *severe* burden only, this figure of tolerance rises to 80%. In group studies, such as this, the assessment of 'objective' burden and 'subjective' burden and of the discrepancy between them would seem to provide a convenient measure of what one might call the general tolerance that prevails in a given community towards the psychiatric patient in the home.

The 'subjective' burden, as we have shown, is much more sensitive to a number of clinical and social factors than is the 'objective' burden. It seems that there was least tolerance for those patients who suffered from epilepsy or showed an organic psychosyndrome, who belonged to the older age-group, who were married persons and who lived in the households of their grown-up children or parents. If they belonged to Social Classes I and II, they were also likely to meet with less tolerance, and the same held if the patient's illness had lasted for from one to two years. A special position was accorded to the schizophrenic patients, who seemed more tolerated than the other diagnostic groups, though there was a fair proportion of 'subjective' burden in these households as well.

The findings in regard to 'subjective' burden beg a number of questions which must at present go unanswered. For instance, one would like to know what the findings would be in the households of patients who had been treated on more conventional lines in a mental hospital, but four-year follow-up studies which would be comparable do not as yet exist. One would further like to know what the figures would be in the households of non-psychiatric patients, who suffer from chronic physical illness only. We know that in our sample 'subjective' burden appeared greater when non-psychiatric illness co-existed with the psychiatric disorder of our patients. A certain amount of similar 'subjective' burden must surely be felt in households when there is a physically sick person to look after, but no psychiatric disorder. So far, however, no figures seem to exist which would make any comparison possible.

Level of Expectation

Any investigation into the household's sense of 'subjective' burden would be incomplete without relating it to the amount of help it had in fact received through the four years. The help offered by social agencies has been examined in an earlier section of this chapter (p. 92), when we subsumed under that heading approximately fifteen statutory and voluntary agencies that provided the bulk of social care in the communities under survey. The question is whether the presence of 'subjective' burden in a household attracted help from any of these agencies and whether the families who complained of 'subjective' burden did receive all the help they expected.

TABLE 44

'Subjective' burden
(by social agency care rendered to the patient or his household)

'Subjective' Burden	*Any Social Agency Care*		*Mental Health Service Care*	
	No	*Yes*	*No*	*Yes*
None	60%	31·5%	56%	26·2%
Some burden	30%	51·1%	33·9%	52·5%
Severe burden	10%	17·4%	10·1%	21·3%
All patients	100%	100%	100%	100%

Table 44 shows that there was a relationship between 'subjective' burden and social agency care. 68·5% of those receiving social agency care had complained of 'subjective' burden, whereas the figure was only 40% for those receiving no such care. Although this difference lies in the expected direction, it is not statistically significant, and only becomes so if severe 'subjective' burden alone is taken into account ($p < 0.01$).

Of all the social agencies the local authority mental health service shows the trend most clearly. In the case of this agency, a significantly larger number of patients receiving social care had also complained of 'subjective' burden, even if this was only moderate. 73·8% of their clients complained of 'subjective' burden, whereas among those whom they did not serve the figure for 'subjective' complaint was only 43% ($p < 0.01$).

Table 44 also shows that although there was a degree of correlation between the sense of 'subjective' burden and social agency care, there seemed to be a proportion of families who were missed by the social agencies, despite the fact that they felt 'subjective' burden; if both severe and slight 'subjective' burden are taken together, the figure is as high as 40% of those who received no social agency care, not even from the mental health services. Particularly striking were the 10% of households who had no social care, yet their 'subjective' burden had been recorded as severe. The reasons for this apparent discrepancy or gap in the co-ordination of the services invite examination. A variety of reasons are likely to have been operative; for instance, social agency care might not have been sensitive enough to need, there were communication breakdowns, and failures perhaps of follow-up after inception into the service; or it could be that the agencies were aware enough of need, but unable to offer any useful help; families could also dislike asking for help or might have little idea where to turn or what was the range of services available. Much as we would have liked to investigate all these points in detail, it was not possible to do this within the framework of the current study as it had been planned. We could only approach the issue broadly.

The views of all the relatives were sought retrospectively at the end of the four years, as to whether they felt that more could have been done to help them. This referred not only to the social agencies, but to the medical services as well.

As one might expect, the families who felt no 'subjective' burden were satisfied and did not think anything more should be done. But of those households who did think more help might

TABLE 45

'Subjective' burden
(by informant's opinion whether
more help should have been given)

'Subjective' Burden	*Should more have been done?*	
	No	*Yes*
None	53·8%	—
Some	38%	80%
Severe	8·2%	20%
Total	100%	100%

have been given, 80% had carried some 'subjective' burden, and in an additional 20% this had been severe.

The startling finding is that 46·2% of the satisfied group, who thought nothing more could have been done, had complained of 'subjective' burden, and 8·2% had felt this as severe. This last group of patients, it is true, would include some who had received social agency care, but apparently this had not been able to ease such burden completely. The fact that severe 'subjective' burden had persisted in this way makes one wonder why these patients were nevertheless satisfied with what had been done.

The figure of 8·2% might be taken as an index of what we might call the 'level of expectation' among our patients' households, i.e. of the amount of help they felt should be available to them in their plight of caring for a psychiatric patient in the home. In our sample this index figure stands at nearly one-tenth, and perhaps it might better be called the index of 'lack of expectation'. It would be interesting to find out whether the figure would be higher or lower in other communities and in particular what it would be in an area served by a conventional mental hospital service. It would also be interesting to know what would be the effect of a high degree of sophistication in the public about the services and in the services themselves as to their responsibilities. The answers to such questions must await further research; as far as we know, no one else has examined these questions as yet and there are no established norms from which to work.

Attitudes to Hospital Service

Informant, Patient, and the Hospital Service After four years it seemed possible that the patients and their households might well have formed some opinions on the extramural service, particularly as this type of service does involve the household to a greater extent and differently from the more conventional hospital service. We tried therefore to learn something about the attitude prevailing among our sample of patients and their relatives.

We undertook this part of the investigation – which again is in the nature of an opinion poll – despite the difficulties which are known to attend this procedure, but we have attempted to avoid too rigid an interpretation of the results.

Desirability of In-patient Admission to Unit The prejudice which exists in wide circles of the public against hospital admission in general and psychiatric hospital admission in particular must surely influence a whole set of attitudes amongst patients and relatives. One notices sometimes with distress that both patients and relatives have to be coerced into the idea of the patient's coming into hospital, even when necessary. It was surprising therefore to find that 88% of our patients' relatives accepted in-patient admission to the unit and only 12% were against it. Table 46 shows that these attitudes were related to the diagnosis of the patient's illness. Where the diagnosis was that of an organic psychosyndrome, admission to the unit was accepted by all as a necessity, whereas the affective psychoses were equally represented in the accepting and rejecting groups. The personality disorders and abnormal psychogenic reactions, however, were much over-represented in the rejecting group. The attitudes of the relatives of the schizophrenic patients showed a similar pattern, though not quite so marked, which is rather surprising. It may be due perhaps to the fact that many of the schizophrenic patients were already sufferers of many years at the time of inception. Nevertheless, the relatively high incidence of families reluctant to see their schizophrenic relatives removed to hospital is surely rather contrary to the expectation of most people. It will be seen therefore that among the one-tenth or so of relatives who felt some reservations about

TABLE 46

Was the informant in favour or against admission to the unit (at time of inception)?

Attitude	*All Cases*	*Organic Psychosyndrome and Epilepsy*	*Affective Psychosis*	*Schizophrenia*	*Personality Disorders and Reactions*	*Others*
Accepting	88%	25%	28%	20%	24%	3%
Against	12%	—	25%	31%	44%	—

in-patient admission to the unit, the diagnostic categories in relation to the patients' illnesses were not randomly distributed, and attitudes appeared influenced by this.

The lapse of time seemed to have little influence on relatives' attitudes. At the end of the four years 16% were still against in-patient admission. The slight difference between this and the percentage given earlier for the attitudes at inception is statistically insignificant. It is thus not surprising that the clinical outcome of the patient's illness had no influence either, remaining the same in all the categories, from recovered, improved through to no change, to worse. However, the aggregate length of time patients actually stayed in the unit did have a certain effect. The relatives of those patients who never were admitted at all to the unit were greatly over-represented among the group who were against admission (45% as compared with 24% in favour of admission). Where patients had stayed up to one month, the representation was almost reversed (20% of those against admission as compared with 39% of those in favour). Once patients had stayed for an aggregate of more than one month, they were almost equally represented in both groups.

Brown *et al.* (1962) showed that if patients received visitors while in hospital, this affected them other than simply comforting them. The number of visits per patient were found to correlate highly with the discharge rate from hospital. This could only be shown to operate in a mental hospital with a rather conservative, restrictive policy of patient care. When this policy was changed to a more permissive one, the correlation disappeared. In this context we were interested to find out what the relatives of patients had felt about visiting at the unit. The majority said they would visit readily, but 6% declared they would regard visiting simply as a duty. No one said that they would not visit at all. With this small figure of 6% any further breakdown was impossible, but there was an interesting relationship with longer-stay patients. It was their relatives who tended most to fall into the category where visiting was undertaken only as a duty.

In general it seemed that a certain adverse attitude towards in-patient admission to the unit tended to come about the longer patients had to stay there, although, of course, the true relationship might be the other way round – namely, patients could stay longer simply because fewer objections had been raised. Table 47 shows the figures.

TABLE 47

What did the relatives feel, at the time of follow-up, about in-patient admission to the unit (by the length of the patient's stay in the unit)?

Relatives' Attitude to Admission	*All Cases*		*Aggregate Length of Stay in the Unit*			
			Nil	*Up to 1 Month*	*2–12 Months*	*13 Months and Over*
In favour	106	84%	24%	39%	24%	14%
Against	20	16%	45%	20%	20%	15%

When we consider the attitudes of the patients themselves, we find a very different situation. As shown in Table 48, half, i.e. 53%, of the patients were at inception reluctant to be admitted, and the proportion had changed only slightly and certainly

TABLE 48

Patient's attitude to in-patient admission to the unit at inception and at follow-up

At Inception	*All Patients*	*At Follow-up*		
		Content	*Reluctant*	*N.A.*
Content	47%	69%	20%	11%
Reluctant	53%	25%	56%	19%
Total	100%	51%	49%	—

insignificantly at follow-up four years later. Further analysis of these figures, however, shows that a change of attitude did take place which is obscured by the overall figures. 20% of those patients who had been content to go into the unit at the beginning had become reluctant at the time of the follow-up, while 25% of those who at first had been reluctant had now changed their minds. Thus the experience of being admitted as an in-patient to the unit did not seem to have the same effect on every patient. About the same proportion of patients were favourably impressed as were put off by this experience. Our own inquiry does not help us to show in detail what was the exact cause of these swings in opinion, but it would clearly be in the interests of the patients and of the service to gain more knowledge about the variables that do in fact affect this situation.

How in retrospect did the relatives evaluate the effects on their households of in-patient admission to the unit? In no case did any relative find that this had made new difficulties for the household. In 44% admission had been felt as making no difference either way, but in 56% it had been experienced as a great relief, particularly where families also reported a sense of severe 'subjective' burden. This group were represented by 16% in the category of great relief, whereas the figure was only 8% where in-patient admissions had made no difference. A similar but much smaller difference was found when a moderate degree of 'subjective' burden had been felt, while the distribution became reversed where families had been free of 'subjective' burden entirely. Grad and Sainsbury (1963) have

TABLE 49

Relatives' opinion: what effect did in-patient admission to the unit have on the household? how did this relate to 'subjective' burden?

Effect on Household	*All Cases*	*'Subjective' Burden*		
		None	*Some*	*Severe*
Made difficulties	—	—	—	—
No effect	44%	51%	41%	8%
Great relief	56%	37%	47%	16%

shown that where in-patient admission is resorted to more frequently, families of patients report greater relief. Our figures would seem to elaborate their findings in showing that in-patient admission is the more likely to be felt as a great relief if the families have developed a sense of 'subjective' burden, although this is by no means invariably so, as can be seen from Table 49.

A proportion of our sample had, of course, never been in-patients at the unit at all. In this instance we asked the relatives if in-patient admission would in their opinion have made difficulties or been a great relief. We found that 10% of the households considered that admission of the patient to the unit would have made difficulties for them, whereas 70% considered that it would have made no difference to them at all. In the 10% who anticipated difficulties the patients (most were male) were all suffering from personality disorders, were from the Burnley area, and tended to come from the larger family group.

A further 20% of the households felt that had the patients been admitted they would have experienced a great relief. Here it seemed that relatives clearly regretted that the patients had not been admitted during the four years. A breakdown of the cases concerned shows that about two-thirds came from the Burnley area and one-third from the Blackpool area; organic psychosyndromes and schizophrenia were the majority diagnoses. Two-thirds were men and one-third were women. This time they came from small family groups and most were married. In these cases it seemed that the unit policy to avoid in-patient admission as much as possible had been felt to be disadvantageous, at least by the relations. Of course, their stated expectations of great relief might not have been fulfilled; nevertheless, that was the extent of the feeling.

Attitude to the Unit's Services To the overall question as to the relatives' attitudes to the unit's service as a whole, 79% replied that they were satisfied; 14% had minor and 7% serious complaints to make. These were not made directly against the new extramural service as a whole, but were more in the nature of the complaints one usually hears in relation to hospitals generally, e.g. quality of food, lack of segregation of patients with different illnesses, particularly of different severity, waiting about for ward rounds, etc. In a few cases the relatives had felt that their side of the situation had not been sufficiently listened to, when, as it seemed to them, they had material points to make, and somehow they felt by-passed. The serious complaints, though relatively few, pointed to what seems to us the key-factor in the success of these extramural services; they concerned schizophrenic patients mainly and those suffering with severe organic psychosyndromes. They amounted to the relatives' sense of being left alone with their problems at times of not infrequent crises. These criticisms do seem directly related to the type and quality of the psychiatric service offered; as an extramural service, one would expect greater ease of communication, of domiciliary visiting and liaison with supporting services; but in these few cases the network of continuing care seemed to have failed.

Brown *et al.* (1962) and Wing *et al.* (1964*b*), among others, have drawn attention to the necessary willingness of relatives to act as nurses and supervisors, and if they receive inadequate support from the psychiatric medical and social services they may well feel unequal to the task and become dissatisfied. Considering that our sample was loaded with cases most likely to give rise to this problem, the number of complaints seems remarkably small. But as such they underline the necessity, not of more hospital care, but of seeing that the efforts of the psychiatric unit and the local health authority are really combined over the individual case, and offer a greater degree of continuity of care than they appear to do at present.

Table 50 shows that the type of illness from which the patient suffered had some relationship with the satisfaction or otherwise which the relative felt in regard to the unit's services. It will be seen that affective psychoses and personality disorders were more highly represented where the relatives were satisfied, whereas organic psychosyndromes and schizophrenia were over-represented among the relatives who had complaints to make. Other factors, such as age of patient, length of morbidity, and length of unit in-patient-stay, had no significant relationship, but not unnaturally complaints tended to be more frequent among those families where the patient's illness proved to have had a poor outcome at the end of the four years.

The patients' own attitudes to the unit services as a whole were not dissimilar to those of their relatives. 80% were satisfied, 19% had minor complaints, and only 1% had severe com-

TABLE 50

What did the relatives feel about the unit?
(by diagnosis of the patient's illness)

Attitude to Unit	*All Cases*	*Diagnoses*				
		Organic Psychosyndrome and Epilepsy	*Schizophrenia*	*Affective Psychosis*	*Personality Disorders and Abnormal Psychogenic Reactions*	*Others*
Satisfied	79%	19%	20%	28%	30%	3%
Minor complaints	14%	30%	40%	13%	17%	—
Major complaints	7%	30%	40%	20%	10%	—

plaints. This latter figure represents two patients only, both from the Burnley catchment area; their complaints referred to rough handling by nursing staff. It must be remembered that they were rather sick patients, and it was also not within our brief to verify individual complaints.

It will be seen that patients were slightly better satisfied than the relatives; their minor complaints were much the same in character, though a fresh objection raised by them was that against psychotherapy, but no complaints were directed against the extramural service as a whole. Rather more complaints came from the older age-group, and, as shown in Table 51, the schizophrenics were relatively over-represented among the complainants, whereas those suffering from personality disorder or abnormal psychogenic reactions were over-represented in the satisfied group. It is, however, noteworthy that a large percentage of schizophrenic patients expressed satisfaction with the unit. The chief complainants appeared to be those suffering with affective psychosis. Other factors, such as the aggregate in-patient-stay in the unit, the length of morbidity, and the clinical outcome did not seem to play any significant role.

Attitudes to Mental Hospital Admission The attitudes of the relatives varied when the question of admission of the patient to mental hospital was raised. Here 22% of the relatives initially objected to this idea, which is a higher percentage than in the case of objections to admissions to the unit (12%). However, just as with the latter, attitudes changed somewhat in the course of the four years and in the same direction, but very much more so. With the adverse attitudes towards admission to the unit, the rise had been insignificant, but in relation to mental hospital admission, the objections rose very significantly from 22% to 52% at the end of the four years ($p < 0{\cdot}001$). We cannot say exactly what this rise denoted nor what it was due to. We do know, however, that most of those who initially had no objection, but later had reservations, were relatives of patients who had never been in-patients of the mental hospital, but had had experience of the unit as such. This would seem to suggest that where an alternative and a more easily accessible one was provided in place of the mental hospital, and where

TABLE 51

What did the patients feel about the unit in general?
(by diagnosis)

Patients' Attitude to Unit	*All Cases*	*Diagnoses*				
		Organic Psychosyndrome and Epilepsy	*Schizophrenia*	*Affective Psychosis*	*Personality Disorders and Abnormal Psychogenic Reactions*	*Others*
Satisfied	80%	4%	20%	28%	47%	1%
Minor complaints	19%	14%	22%	39%	25%	—
Major complaints	1%	—	50%	50%	—	—

relatives had become familiarized with it, they came to prefer this alternative when in-patient treatment was necessary for the patient. This appears to be a fairly clear indication of the success of this administrative policy. On the other hand, with the smaller group who had had experience of mental hospital, the above change in attitude might have been to a certain extent directly related to the unpleasantness of the mental hospital itself; the hospital was more difficult to reach and patients' complaints about having to be there might make the

TABLE 52

What did the relatives feel about mental hospital admission at inception and at follow-up?

Attitude to Mental Hospital Admission		*All Cases*	*Social Class of Patient*		
			I and II	*III*	*IV and V*
At inception	In favour	78%	22%	34%	44%
	Against	22%	34%	55%	11%
4 years later	In favour	48%	25%	47%	28%
	Against	52%	19%	54%	27%

situation more difficult for the relatives. From Table 52 it can be seen that at inception the prejudice against mental-hospital admission seemed rather more prevalent in Social Classes I and II, but at the end of the four-year period the difference disappears.

The patients themselves were against mental-hospital admission to a much larger extent at the time of inception than were the relatives. 44% expressed reluctance. During the four years there was again a rise in the figure, but not so steep as among the relatives. 59% of the patients at follow-up showed reluctance about the idea of admission, which is only slightly higher than among the informants. The older age-group were slightly but not significantly more adverse to admission; social class did not affect the situation, neither initially nor at follow-up. Rich and poor, educated and uneducated, dislike mental-hospital admission equally when it comes to going there themselves.

Attitudes to Treatment Received The relatives were also asked whether in retrospect the actual treatment received by the patient had seemed to them appropriate. 88% felt that this had indeed been so, but 12% were dissatisfied. The age of the patients did not seem to have any influence on this particular attitude. Among the diagnostic groupings, it was the organic psychosyndromes, the epilepsies, and to a lesser extent the schizophrenics where misgivings had been felt. Neither the duration of the psychiatric morbidity nor of non-psychiatric ill-health during the four years was significant, but the relatives of those patients who died were very largely represented among the group who thought treatment had not been appropriate. It seemed that patients suffering from their terminal illness had in the eyes of their relatives not altogether received the treatment expected. An important question is whether the relatives' critical attitudes were in any way related to the length of time spent in mental hospital by the patient, but although the longer-stay patients were slightly over-represented in the dissatisfied group of relatives, the differences were not significant. It was also perhaps interesting to note that the relatives of those patients who had committed suicide were not to be found among the complainant group.

Could More Have Been Done? Finally, the question was put to the relatives, whether they thought more could have been done by the medical or social services to help them and the patient throughout the four years. 91% said, 'No'; 9% said, 'Yes'. This 9% comprised a total of fourteen cases. A more detailed look at this group showed that the majority of the patients (twelve) were under sixty years of age. In three cases they were suffering from organic psychosyndromes, in two cases from epilepsy, in eight cases from schizophrenia, and in one case from personality disorder. Six of the patients had stayed more than three months as unit in-patients, and another three had stayed from one to three months. Five of them had not been in-patients at all. None of them had had mental hospital experience. All their families had complained of 'subjective' burden; in ten cases of moderate burden, in four cases of severe burden. The findings are not particularly revealing. They show that most of the dissatisfied relatives belonged to those patient-groups that had been found vulnerable, in other respects dissatisfied, but they formed a small minority of these. When the patient-group as a whole was asked whether they felt more could have been done for them over the four years, only 5% thought this might have been so.

Conclusions

On the whole, therefore, the general picture given here is of a large degree of satisfaction on the part of patients and relatives, and there would seem to be some indication that in-patient treatment at the psychiatric unit became accepted and preferred by the majority of them to mental-hospital treatment. The various attitudes elicited here have perhaps raised more questions than could be answered at this stage; they certainly show that a small but not insignificant number of relatives and patients did not feel that sufficient help had been given to them, although much the same type of care and service had been extended to them as to others who had not complained; certainly some of the patients in this group posed serious and intransigent problems, as the following may illustrate:

The patient was a woman in late middle life, living with her husband of the same age. She had suffered for many years from an organic psychosyndrome. At the time of inception at the unit her illness was well advanced (G.P.I.), and she had had previously some years of mental-hospital treatment. Her husband had left work before his retiring age to look after her, as she was extremely difficult to manage and incontinent, but he seemed to have deemed it his duty to do this. He had become himself tense, diffident, depressed, and hostile. The patient's illness was reaching its terminal state, and she died in the course of two years. The unit's service had been one of consultation only at out-patient's and return to the care of her general practitioner. Thereafter the couple appear to have become isolated to what seemed the detriment of the husband's own health and other social relationships.

CHAPTER IV

Special Findings

INTRODUCTION

Although this largely extramural type of management of an unselected group of psychiatric patients seemed to work well on the whole from the point of view of patients, relatives, and the supporting services, there were, as we have seen, a small number of patients to whom this did not altogether apply. Amongst the unselected intake of the units as such they only formed a minority, and they were by no means a homogeneous group. The question arises, however, whether there are in fact recognizable sub-groups of patients in which failures of management may turn from a small minority into a sizeable one, or even into a majority. In other words, do we find any special groups among psychiatric patients for whom an extramural type of management is particularly unsuited or less suited than for most other patients?

Two groups which would immediately come under suspicion are the schizophrenic patients and the elderly. Illnesses in both these groups tend to be of a chronic and often intractable nature, and are likely to create difficulties in social adjustment. This suspicion will occur to any experienced clinician. He may well argue that, while it is feasible for psychiatric patients in general to be managed successfully in the community, so that our findings so far do not appear incredible, these two particular groups are likely to produce problems which so far have not been conspicuous in our findings because the patients, being relatively small in number, have been submerged in the picture of the group as a whole.

With this possibility in mind, we extracted from our total sample all cases falling into these two groups, and examined our findings once more as they applied to each in turn. Not only does this test the question of whether these two groups contain a larger proportion of failures, but it will throw light on factors which bring about failures or success, so that when weaknesses become apparent, measures can be taken to remedy them.

(I) SCHIZOPHRENIC PATIENTS

Our sample contained sixty-two schizophrenic patients. This represented 1·39 per 10,000 population, and the proportion was the same for both the catchment areas. The two units were studied separately, but, as findings were so similar, we have presented them together.

The Patients

The general characteristics of the schizophrenic group were as follows:

Sex and Age The group contained twenty-nine males (47%) and fifty-three females (53%), which was very similar to the total population of the units. It represents 1·39 per 10,000 male population in the area and 1·41 of the female population. The rates are higher than those given by Shepherd (1957), who found that first-admission schizophrenics to mental hospital in the years 1945–7 amounted to 0·52 males and 0·54 females per 10,000 population. It must be remembered that Shepherd only counted those schizophrenics who were admitted as in-patients, whereas our sampling also included those who remained as out-patients. The comparison certainly shows that the units did not have a smaller number of schizophrenics to deal with than other psychiatric services elsewhere. Unlike the clinic sample as a whole, the majority of the schizophrenics were in the under-sixty-year age-group; only four patients (6%), all women, were in the over-sixty-year age-group, three of them over seventy years of age. In the total sample the over-sixty-year age-group comprised 33%. In the under-sixty-year age-group among the schizophrenics the sexes were fairly equally represented, which was again very similar to the general group.

Social Class

The largest number of patients fell into R.G. Social Class III (46%); the next largest into Classes II and IV, with 12·9% each. 3·2% were found in Class I. This social-class distribution was very similar to what had been found for the sample as a whole, as shown in Table 12, with the exception of Class V, which, with 19·4%, contained slightly more schizophrenics at the expense of Classes II and IV, a not unexpected finding. The social-class distribution in relation to the catchment area is not known, as the relevant census tract for 1961 has not yet appeared.

Education

Educational attainment was as follows: the majority (66·1%) had the equivalent of secondary modern education; 19·4% had had grammar school education; 1·6% had been to special schools for the educationally subnormal. In 12·9% no information was available. These figures are very similar to those found for the psychiatric sample as a whole, as shown in Table 11.

Civil Status

As is common with schizophrenic patients, the majority were single people (62%). Not more than 6% were known to be living alone at inception. These figures contrast sharply with what we found for the psychiatric sample as a whole (Table 6), which shows that only 28% were single persons and 72% were ever married ($p < 0{\cdot}001$). This difference is highly significant and confirms that our sample was typical for schizophrenics in general, who are known to contain a high proportion of single persons.

Mobility

The schizophrenic group showed a high incidence of geographical mobility. Only 35·6% were indigenous to their catchment area. Of the 'immigrant' group (46·7%), most had come from elsewhere in the United Kingdom, and only two patients had come from abroad. In 17·7% reliable information was unobtainable, but even if this group were added to the indigenous group, immigrant numbers would still be noticeably high. Yet the findings are not so very different from the sample as a whole, the figures for which have been given in Table 10.

Management of Patients

It will be remembered that only newly incepted patients were included in our research sample. It has been mentioned before, however, that this did not mean that patients had not received treatment elsewhere before they came to the units. In fact, the figures for the schizophrenic patients were nearly three times as high for the psychiatric sample as a whole (Table 16). 50% had had psychiatric treatment elsewhere either because they were resident in some other part of the country or because treatment had been given in a more distant past, before the units had opened; but as regards duration of their illness, the figures were very similar to the total sample (Table 15). In 42%, the illness had already lasted for more than two years before the patients presented themselves at the unit, and in another 28% the illness had lasted for considerably more than six months. Only 30% had been ill for less than this. Thus in 70% the illness was well established at inception and both units were dealing with a largely chronic group.

Most of these were first seen as unit out-patients and a few, mainly the elderly, on domiciliary visits. After this first inception, however, they were dealt with in the following manner, which was not much different from what happened in the unselected group of the total sample (see p. 57): the largest group (55%) were admitted as in-patients (48·5% to the unit beds, 6·5% to mental hospital beds). The patients admitted to mental hospital were all from the Blackpool unit, which, as we have shown, was suffering from a shortage of unit beds. A further 6·5% became day-patients at the units, while a surprisingly large number (38·5%) were not admitted as in- or day-patients, but remained as out-patients. This may be due to the fact that many were indeed chronic sufferers on first inception and vigorous in-patient treatment had already been tried in the past, perhaps with but limited effect. If this is taken into account, one can see that the unit policy of liberal initial in-patient admission was pursued as much with the schizophrenic group of patients as with the rest of the sample, and there can be no talk of a policy that 'keeps patients out of hospital at all costs' – a misinformed statement not uncommonly levied against extramural care.

Furthermore, irrespective of whether patients become in-patients or remained as out-patients, they came under some form of active treatment. Thus 42·9% of our group receivep electro-convulsive treatment with or without pharmaca; another 48% had drug treatment alone (mainly the promazine drugs) and only 8·1% underwent some form of psychotherapy or occupational therapy alone. Something in fact was offered for every patient.

We will now look at the management of the patients during the four-year period as a whole (including the initial phase). Although, as we have seen, the initial rate of in-patient admission was high, relatively little time was in fact spent in hospital at any point. Most patients had several in-patient admissions during the four years – sometimes to the unit, sometimes to the mental hospital. Taking these separately, we find that about 60% became unit in-patients, which is very similar to the figure for the group as a whole (66%), and 37% mental-hospital in-patients, which is twice as many as for the group as a whole (19%), as can be seen from Table 20. Some patients, of course, fell into both categories, at one stage of their illness entering the unit, at another being admitted to the mental hospital. The relatively high admission rate to mental hospital was mainly due to the situation in Blackpool. In the Burnley area the figures were much smaller (6%). The differences between the schizophrenic and the general psychiatric sample remains consistent in the two units.

Because of the general complexity of the pattern of repeated admission and readmission to unit or mental hospital over the four years, we chose to present the data in summary form. We found that only 14·5% of our schizophrenics had never been in-patients of any kind during the period; 66·2% of them had been in-patients at one time or another. Of the remaining 19·3% some had died during the four-year period and others were untraceable.

In regard to the 66·2% who had been in-patients, we sought to find out how extensive the hospitalization had been. We established the 'total hospital time' – that is, the aggregate length of time spent as in-patient, in unit or mental hospital, irrespective of whether this was continuous or the sum of several short spells distributed over the whole four years.

If we look at this 'total hospital time', we find that 21% of our schizophrenic group spent a total of less than three months as in-patients (5% of the follow-up period), and most of this had been at inception. Another 35% spent from four to twelve months as in-patients (6–25% of the total period); a further group, amounting to 4·8% of the patients, spent from one to two years (25–50% of the period). These could be regarded as medium-stay patients, leaving only another 4·8% who stayed for two years or more (over 50% of the period). The really long-stay patient group, therefore, composed less than 5% of the schizophrenic group, of whom the large majority (95%) spent two years or more within their own community. 35·5%, moreover, were never admitted at all or only for a few weeks, usually in the initial period. Compared with the psychiatric sample as a whole, there was a tendency amongst the schizophrenic patients to spend somewhat more time as in-patients, although the differences were not as marked as might be expected (see Table 22).

As many studies reported in the literature give a point-prevalence figure at the end of the specific follow-up period of such patients, we give our own findings here, although to our mind they are not nearly as illuminating as figures which show the four-year follow-up longitudinally. Only 9·6% of our schizophrenic patients were at the time actually in hospital. This compares very favourably with the figure (27·4%) given by Mandelbrote *et al.* (1961*a*), which was nearly three times as high. These workers were also investigating a community-orientated service, but based on a mental, not a general hospital. In other more conventional types of psychiatric service, the figure is very much higher.

The general pattern which seems to emerge from this investigation of length of hospital stay shows that the schizophrenics as a group spent more time as in-patients than did the total sample of unselected psychiatric patients (see Table 22).

81% of these latter were never hospitalized over the four years, or, if so, stayed for less than three months, as compared with 56·5% of the schizophrenics. Nevertheless, the schizophrenics did remain in the community to a very large extent, and the difference from what was customary for this type of patient in the past is most striking. Shepherd (1957), when studying the figures for the years 1953 to 1955, showed that the great majority of schizophrenics once admitted to mental hospital remained there for at least five years. Compared with that, our own findings certainly indicate a new departure in the management of this serious condition.

Effects on the Patient and His Environment

For the first time we have investigated an unselected annual intake of schizophrenic patients new to this particular service, who spent most of the following four-year period in the community. We had an opportunity, therefore, to examine to what extent this affected the course of their illness and their general social adjustment. It would seem that the new type of management could have had a profound influence on these patients no less than on their environment.

Morbidity

26% of the group continued ill for less than one year; another 7·2% for less than two years. 46·5%, however, remained ill for two or more years out of the whole four-year period. Information on the remainder was incomplete. The point-prevalence morbidity at the end of the period was as follows: 27% had recovered, another 27·5% had improved, but 16·2% had failed to improve or were worse. 9·7% had died. In 19% reliable information could not be obtained. These figures indicate a very high amount of morbidity both during the four-year period and cross-sectionally at the end of the period as a whole. As shown previously in Table 26, the morbidity rate in schizophrenia was considerably higher than in the other diagnostic groups, with the exception of the organic psychosyndromes and epilepsy.

Just under 10% of the patients died at very varying points

during the four years, and were therefore excluded from the general evaluation of our results. Two patients died by suicide, both under sixty years of age, one male and one female. In the other four patients death was due to non-psychiatric accidental causes (e.g. cancer, nephritis, diabetes, etc.). Two of these patients were over sixty years of age. The death-rate for the psychiatric sample as a whole will be found discussed in Section III of this chapter (pp. 193ff.).

Comparison with the morbidity rate in other studies is scarcely possible, which is frustrating. For one thing, there simply are no studies that give a periodic prevalence rate at all and available investigations show a point-prevalence rate at the end of longer or shorter follow-up periods. On this rather blunt method of assessing outcome, our own findings are fairly similar to two follow-up studies from the Maudsley Hospital, one by Shepherd (1958) and one by Leiberman *et al.* (1957). In both groups (one after five years, one after three years) 30–1% of the patients had recovered and 31% had improved. The rest were unchanged or worse. In our own group 27% recovered, 27·5% improved. Mandelbrote *et al.* (1961 *a* and *b*) followed up patients, who were managed on an extramural basis from a mental hospital over a four-year period. They seemed to have slightly poorer results. They simply divided their group into 'well' and 'not well'. They found at the end of the period 41·6% 'well', similar to Wing *et al* (1964*b*), who studied short-stay patients discharged from mental hospital after one year. The latter found 41% showing 'minimal disorder', the others were more seriously ill by that time. These comparisons suggest that consistent management on an extramural basis from the time of inception of the patient does not in itself change the prevalence of morbidity in schizophrenic patients. Our findings are a little better than those for patients treated in mental hospital, and they are very similar to those for patients who have been managed from a psychiatric teaching hospital – namely, the Maudsley Hospital, London.

Work Adjustment

In view of the high morbidity rate, one would expect a good deal of invalidism among our patients. We tried to assess this by looking at the employment figures, having excluded those who had reached retirement age and all women who were full-time housewives. This gave a working population of forty-three patients. Of this group 41% were working for at least three years (75%) of the period; 21% had worked for periods of from one to three years; 38% had been almost completely unemployed throughout. Comparison with Table 28 shows that there was more unemployment than with the psychiatric sample as a whole, and if diagnostic groupings are compared (Table 28) there was more unemployment with schizophrenia than with the rest, with the exception of the organic psychosyndromes and epilepsy, where the figures were very similar. Employment as such is a considerable measure of social adjustment. Many schizophrenics left with a defect state can return to work, but often of a different, usually lower quality. As regards this qualitative change in the employment record, we found a decline in social class in 17% of the working group. Of these who moved down, all were men, belonging originally to Social Classes II or III, and all ended in Social Class V. Only one patient, a woman, had moved up from Class III to Class II. Two patients had had to seek sheltered employment. One woman gave up work altogether and became a housewife, but remained active in that capacity.

TABLE 53

Schizophrenia
Aggregate duration of employment

Proportion of Follow-up Time employed	*Mandelbrote's Extramural Mental Hospital Service* (1 *year F.U.*)	*Wing's Experimental Hospital In-patients* (1 *year F.U.*)	*Present Study General Hospital Psychiatric Unit* (4 *years F.U.*)
0– 25%	15·2%	48·2%	41%
25– 75%	5·8%	18%	21%
75–100%	62·5%	34%	38%

Table 53 gives an approximate comparison of findings as between our own group and two other studies, though in both these latter the follow-up time was only one year as contrasted with our four years. It was impossible to match the employment categories exactly, so that the comparison can only be an approximate one.

If work adjustment decreases with length of follow-up period, Mandelbrote's figures would seem to suggest a worse outcome than ours, though the group of patients and the type of management are reasonably comparable with what we had in our own study. However, in Mandelbrote's case the psychiatric unit was not situated in a general hospital, but in a mental hospital, and perhaps this difference exerted some influence on the type of patient referred in the first place. Possibly the rather higher in-patient disposal at inception and the longer hospital stay also had some influence.

The figures in Wing's study appear at first more in line with ours, but, as they only cover a one-year follow-up period, they are in fact rather worse. A similar study by Shepherd (1958) of ex-patients has been omitted here, as the information on employment is too fragmentary to be evaluated; he merely states that '50 per cent. of those who had not recovered had worked for 50 per cent. of the 5-year follow-up period'.

At the end of the follow-up period we found a 40% point prevalence of unemployed, which is much the same figure as Mandelbrote *et al.* found at the end of one year (42%). They, however, did not follow up all their cases and they excluded those patients who were still in hospital, whereas in our case this group were included in our figures and recorded as unemployed. We cannot therefore adjust the two scales.

Although we had excluded full-time housewives from the above employment analysis, we nevertheless looked at their general competence as a group. We found that four of them had had the capacity to cope with home duties for at least three years; one woman had coped up to two years, while three women had been entirely incapacitated throughout the whole four-year period. The absolute number of schizophrenic housewives is very small, but the figures, for what they are worth, indicate that their illness did affect work capacity to a not inconsiderable extent.

The general picture of work adjustment in our schizophrenic group of patients cannot be considered as altogether satisfactory, as might be expected from the morbidity rate, that was higher than in the total sample. Nevertheless, the completely unemployed were just over one-third of the group, and two-thirds at least made some working contribution, 41% for a major part of the time, even if at a lower level of skill in some cases. Considering the serious nature of the illness, this is in some ways not a bad result, particularly if we compare it with what used to happen in previous years to schizophrenic patients, who tended to spend most of their time in mental hospital once the illness had struck (Shepherd, 1957; Norris, 1959).

Use of Other Services

General Practitioner

As the patients spent relatively little time in hospital, despite the high degree of morbidity, the question inevitably arose whether they required the help of other types of care, medical or social. It would, for instance, not be unexpected if some extra load fell on to the general practitioner. We tried to assess this by counting the contacts which took place between the patient and the general practitioner during the four-year period, irrespective of whether the patient had called at the surgery or the doctor had come to the house. As this had to be assessed in retrospect, a certain number of cases had to be discounted because the information was unobtainable or unreliable. Of the forty-three patients on whom full data could be obtained, 22% had had no contact with their general practitioner throughout the entire period. Another 57% had had less than one contact in six months; only 27% could claim two or more contacts in six months.

Table 54 shows that the call on the general practitioner services depended very much on the degree of morbidity during the four years. Of those patients who were ill for under two years, only 7% had more than two contacts in six months, but where the illness had lasted over the two years, the figure rises to 37%. Though the difference seems considerable, the absolute numbers were small and the difference does not reach statistical significance.

Our figures can be compared with those reported by Mandelbrote *et al.* (1961*a* and *b*). In a group of schizophrenic patients managed on extramural lines he found that 28%

TABLE 54

Schizophrenia
Frequency of general practitioner consultations according to the aggregate duration of mental ill health

Duration of Mental Ill Health	General Practitioner Consultations			
	None	Up to 1 Contact in 6 Months	2 or more Contacts in 6 Months	Total
Less than 2 years	23%	70%	7%	100%
More than 2 years	21%	42%	37%	100%
Total	22%	57%	21%	100%

received drugs from their general practitioners while out of hospital; this comes very close to our figure of 25% (patients having two or more contacts in six months). Not all Mandelbrote's patients, however, were followed up for the full four years, as in our case. Our figures are also similar to those of Wing *et al.* (1964*b*), who followed up their group of discharged mental hospital schizophrenic patients after one year. They then found 28% had regular contact with their general practitioner. Occasional contact showed a figure of 44%; in our own group this was 54%. Such comparisons have to be cautious, but our results here seem fairly in line with what befalls the patient in other studies.

On an average our schizophrenics had 4·5 contacts with their general practitioners per annum. This appears slightly less than the national average for general practice (Logan *et al.*, 1958), which has been calculated at six contacts per annum. It is also less than the average for all types of psychiatric patients, which was found to be approximately twelve contacts per annum. Other comparisons between diagnostic groups are shown in Table 30.

It seems therefore that far from being any extra burden on the general practitioner service, our particular group of schizophrenics called for appreciably less help from general practice than did the psychiatric sample as a whole, or the average of the general population.

Non-psychiatric Hospital Services

Psychiatric hospitalization having been avoided to a large extent, one might wonder whether some form of 'hidden' hospitalization might not have taken its place. This might be possible, for instance, if such patients drifted into general medical or geriatric beds (Kidd, 1962*b*). In fact, only four patients in this group were admitted to general medical beds in the course of the four years. The reasons for this were definitely *not* psychiatric, and all the patients were short-stay only (four weeks in two cases, under twelve weeks in the other two cases).

Social Services

One might also expect that with this extramural manageme n the social services might become quite heavily engaged and patients rely on more extensive support from them. Very few studies so far have set out to assess the amount of social help actually given or required and there is room for some clarification. Table 55 gives a list of the statutory and voluntary agencies included in our survey. In each case their involvement during the four years was recorded. When this was finally assessed, we found, contrary to our expectation, that the contribution made by these agencies was relatively small. The only one that could be said to have been used to any major extent was the local authority Mental Health Service, which assisted in 44% of the cases. This seems appropriate, as this service is visualized as the key social service for psychiatric patients. The National Assistance Board supported 16% and the Ministry of Labour helped some 26%. The other agencies, including the voluntary ones, were never involved with more than 6% of the patients, and in most cases very much less than this. With the psychiatric sample as a whole (Tables 32 *a* and *b*), the same agencies seem involved but to a lesser extent, e.g. the figure for the Mental Health Services was 31%, for the National Assistance Board and the Ministry of Labour, 12%.

TABLE 55

Schizophrenia
The social agencies

Statutory Agencies	*Amount of Usage*	
Mental Health Service	27	44%
Health Visitor Service	1	2%
Home Help Service	1	2%
District Nurse Service	—	
Social Welfare Department	1	2%
Housing Department	—	
National Assistance Board	10	16%
Ministry of Pensions and National Insurance	1	2%
Ministry of Labour	16	26%
Children's Department	1	2%
Probation Service or prison	2	3%
Any other agency	4	6%
Voluntary Agencies		
Place of work	3	5%
Church or chapel	1	2%
Other voluntary organizations	—	—

One patient or household, of course, might have used several agencies. If therefore all social agency care for the schizophrenic patients is brought together, irrespective of the specific type of agency care involved, the following picture emerges: Of the fifty-one cases where full information was available, 37% had received no social agency care whatever, and 41% had occasional care, which meant that only 22% had received anything like constant or periodic care. Table 33 shows that these figures are slightly lower than in the psychiatric sample as a whole.

Neither the patient's sex, age, social class, duration of illness, geographical mobility, nor type of household seemed to have any influence on the amount of social care received, and none of the statutory services appeared to have exceeded the ordinary provision of occasional or more regular, routine help.

As there are no comparable studies that survey the field of social care as a whole, and therefore have the same scope as ours, overall comparison with other investigations cannot be made. We can, however, compare a number of individual aspects. For instance, Mandelbrote *et al.* (1961 *a* and *b*) found that the National Assistance Board rendered help in 30·9% of their sample, which is considerably more than 16% in our group. On the other hand, the Ministry of Labour gave help to only 5·9% of their cases, but was called upon by 26% of ours. Wing *et al.* (1964) found that their ex-mental patients were helped to an even higher extent by this agency – namely, 38%. In this case the patients underwent an active programme of rehabilitation; for instance, the Disablement Rehabilitation Officer alone was involved with 22% of the cases. In spite of this, however, Wing's group showed a much higher readmission rate than ours. Strangely enough, the agency most involved in our case (the local authority Mental Health Service) was mentioned neither by Mandelbrote and his team, nor by Wing and his. Our figure of 44% usage of this service seems close to that reported by Waters *et al.* (1965), who also studied a group of schizophrenic patients discharged from a mental hospital. They were looking mainly at patients who had been in mental hospital a long time, as opposed to Wing's sample, who had been mainly short-stay patients. But, in common with Wing's sample, the patients had also undergone an intensive rehabilitation programme and were carefully selected and prepared for discharge from hospital. The local authority Mental Health Service was called upon by about half of these patients, but unfortunately strict comparison is not possible.

Mandelbrote *et al.* (1961*b*) mention the Housing Department, which extended help to 5·3%, but in our group there was no call on the Housing Department at all. Help given by voluntary agencies seemed as small in Mandelbrote's group as in our own. In their sample 5·9% were supported by social clubs, but it is not clear under whose auspices these were run – by the hospital, local authority, or voluntary organization.

Finally, 37% of our patients had no social care whatsoever. This figure is rather similar to the 48·9% of Mandelbrote *et al.* and the 29% of Waters *et al.* Both these latter studies concluded, however, that there were a fair number of cases where social care had been objectively indicated but not in fact given. In our group the subjective need as experienced by the patient's household seemed rather low and we studied the question in some detail, relating the social agency care given to families where on the one hand there was 'objective' burden and on the other where 'subjective' burden had been felt. We found that whether social agency care was given or not was more closely related to the existence of 'subjective' need than to the presence of 'objective' burden as such.

The question of how great a need there was for more social agency care to be increased is a hard one to answer. As many as 19% of the patients' households thought that more should have been done, though the patients themselves only thought so to the extent of 7%. In the general psychiatric group, it was 9% of the relatives and 5% of the patients who took up this attitude. Waters *et al.* (1965) have drawn attention to the fact that help is more usually directed towards the patient individually, whereas the patient's household tends to get lost sight of, even with good out-patient care. We cannot say whether this was the case in our own group. If so, this might account for the greater amount of dissatisfaction expressed by the households. That families looking after schizophrenic patients feel more need for this kind of support than the families of patients with other psychiatric illnesses is not perhaps surprising.

Lack of social agency care may have more tangible effects. For instance, it may lead to a series of crises requiring readmission. In that respect Waters *et al.* (1965) found that readmission to hospital (the failure of extramural management) did not occur more often when no social agency care had been given than where it had. This aspect would certainly seem to call for much more detailed studies. Crises leading to readmission may not be related to social agency care as such and may rather depend on other shortcomings in the service. Wing *et al.* (1964*b*) found that many readmissions were linked with failure of patients to take their drugs regularly, but this might perhaps be prevented to a certain extent by a closer follow-up – for instance, the mental health department might create a better liaison between patients, their general practitioner, and the out-patient services. Although the amount of overall social agency care in our own group was no greater than that reported in other studies, and in many respects less intensive, our patients, nevertheless, had the smallest readmission rate.

The role of the social agencies in the management of schizophrenic patients leaves much to be investigated. Our findings definitely suggest that the extramural type of management of these chronic patients had not placed an undue burden at this stage on the general practitioner, other hospitals, or the social agencies. The fact that, despite the relatively little social care which our group of patients received, they did in some respects rather better than those investigated in other follow-up studies, suggests that extramural care based on a general hospital psychiatric unit does make its contribution to the successful management of this type of case.

Effects on the Household

Of even greater interest than the effect which chronic schizophrenics may have on the supporting services when they are kept largely out of hospital is the possible burden which may devolve on their household. To have a member of the household suffering from this disease, even in its attenuated form, must inevitably create burden and distress on other family members. This might well be so, even if the patients find some kind of employment. A large proportion of our schizophrenics (nearly half) were not described as recovered or improved, and it seemed as if a considerable burden might have arisen over the four years. In trying to assess this we used the same methods as described earlier, again observing the 'objective' effects of the patient's illness and the 'subjective' burden felt by the household.

Table 56 shows the amount of actual adverse effect on the households of the patients. It must be remembered that many of these effects occurred only periodically and there might have been long periods in the four years when they did not apply. If we look at each individual category of burden and compare the findings for schizophrenic patients with those for the total psychiatric sample irrespective of diagnosis (Table 34), we find that there was not much difference, except as regards the financial status of the patient. This seemed to have suffered in nearly twice as many cases in the schizophrenic group (30%) as in the general sample (16·5%). It would appear in line with the higher degree of unemployment among the schizophrenics and

TABLE 56

Schizophrenia
Adverse effects on household

Type of Objective Burden caused by Patient's Illness	*Households affected*
Financial:	
Financial status of patient or of household has suffered	30%
Any member of household has lost earnings	7%
Any member of household had to start going out to work	5%
Health:	
Physical strain caused by patient's illness to any member of the household	—
Poor health in any member of the household	16%
Children:	
Separation of children under 16 from their parents	12%
Distress in children under 16	2%
General:	
Disruption of the life of any member of the household	some, 34% much, 8% } 42%

the larger number of them who had declined in social class during the four years. We also find that in twice as many cases members of the household had suffered in health as a direct result of the patient's illness (16% in the schizophrenic group as compared with 6·9% in the general group).

Table 57 records the 'objective' burden on the household as constituted by disturbing behaviour on the part of the patients. A quick comparison with Table 35, which records the findings in the total sample, shows that among the schizophrenics this type of burden tended to appear in very many more cases. This is what we might well expect, and again reflects the high morbidity rate, also the particularly disturbing aspects of schizophrenic behaviour.

The highest discrepancy with the total sample was in category 11 – 'other unusual behaviour' – which was noted in 41% of schizophrenics, as against 25·5% of the total sample. The other

TABLE 57

Schizophrenia
'Objective' burden due to disturbing behaviour

	Constant or Periodic	*Occasional*
1. Noisy or wandering at night	10%	3%
2. Dangerous to themselves or to others	20%	5%
3. Unacceptable sexual behaviour	—	—
4. Generally restless, noisy, or talkative	18%	2%
5. Unresponsive	10%	5%
6. Apparently wilfully unco-operative	25%	7%
7. Used odd speech, or expressed unusual ideas	38%	10%
8. Hypochondriasis	—	3%
9. Requiring nursing or physical care	2%	3%
10. Demanding excessive companionship	5%	3%
11. Other unusual behaviour	41%	8%
12. Any type of disturbing behaviour	60%	

categories, however, were also more frequent for the schizophrenic group, except the category 'need for nursing care'. The higher incidence here for the total sample was very likely due to the fact that on average it held a higher age-group and contained a large number of organic psychosyndromes and non-psychiatric illnesses.

If this combined 'objective' burden is considered, we find that 31% had not caused any type of 'objective' burden at all, whereas 69% had created some such type of difficulty for their households. In the total psychiatric sample the corresponding figures were 44·3% and 55·7%, which indicates that there was a tendency for the schizophrenic group to have more serious effects upon their households.

Whereas in the total psychiatric sample the sex of the patient did not seem to make any difference to the results, among the schizophrenics the male patients did create rather more 'objective' burden. Table 58 shows that age also played a part.

TABLE 58

Schizophrenia
'Combined objective' burden
(by age of patient)

Ages	15–29 *Years*	30–39 *Years*	40–49 *Years*	50–59 *Years*	60 *Years and Over*	*All Ages*
No burden	21%	26·1%	26·4%	16%	11%	100%
Burden	51%	23%	14%	7%	5%	100%
Total	42%	24%	18%	10%	6%	100%

The younger schizophrenic tended to create more burden. The most marked difference occurs in the fifteen to twenty-nine-year and thirty to thirty-nine-year age-groups (51% and 23% respectively). Again, in the total sample such age discrepancies did not become apparent. The high incidence of 'objective' burden in the households of the younger patients, predominantly male, was perhaps due rather more to the financial loss suffered as a result of unemployment than to their disturbing behaviour. The civil status of the patient did not seem to affect the 'objective' burden among the schizophrenic group any more than for the sample population as a whole. It was in both cases unrelated.

In view of Brown *et al.*'s (1962) findings that ex-hospital patients maintain a better social adjustment if they live away from their parents, this aspect was also considered. Table 59 shows that there seemed more 'objective' burden in the parental homes than in the others, and it was greater in the conjugal home than if the patient lived with other kin or alone. The differences, however, are not significant, even if they are in line with Brown's contention that emotional involvement between patient and household has a deleterious effect. It is interesting, moreover, to see from Table 36 that this result did not apply to our psychiatric patient group as a whole. At first glance, therefore, there seems support for the further contention of Waters *et al.* (1965) and Kelley (1964) that the type of household to

TABLE 59

Schizophrenia
'Combined objective' burden
(by type of household)

Type of Patient's Home	*With Parents*	*With Spouse*	*With Other Kin*	*Living Alone or at No Fixed Abode*	*Total*
No burden	40%	30%	20%	10%	100%
Burden	56%	32%	12%	10%	100%

which patients return does not after all have any significant effect on the subsequent course of the illness nor on the patients' social adjustment. Social class seemed to have no relation to the 'objective' burden. Duration of morbidity, highly related to the combined 'objective' burden in the total sample, did not seem to have the same relationship in the schizophrenic patients; there was a trend, it is true – duration of illness for more than two years meant heavier 'objective' burden—but the differences did not reach significance.

'Subjective' Burden

Whether there was any 'subjective' burden or not depended on whether there had been some informant who had stayed in the household through the period and was now available for interview. These conditions were present in forty-three cases. In only 9% of these did the relatives report severe 'subjective' burden; in 51% they reported some burden, while in 40% there was no 'subjective' complaint at all. Slight differences in sex of the patient and duration of illness, etc., did occur, but in no case were these differences statistically significant. There seemed a tendency for male patients (61%) to create 'subjective' burden rather more frequently than the female patients (40%), particularly as regards a moderate degree of burden. Severe 'subjective' burden was in fact felt less in the schizophrenic group (9%) than in the total sample, where it applied to 19·6% (Table 39).

We find, therefore, that the overall figure for 'subjective' complaint among the households of schizophrenic patients was 60%, i.e. the proportion of households where there was *any* such complaint. This compares with 54% in the total psychiatric group. The figure for any 'objective' burden was 69%, which also was somewhat higher than the figure reported for the total psychiatric patient group (58·7%, $p < 0{\cdot}05$).

Relationship between 'Objective' and 'Subjective' Burden

In order to discover the relationships between these two types of burden, we had to work on a reduced total of forty-three cases, in which full information on both aspects could be elicited. We found that in this group a higher proportion of households (81%) carried 'objective' burden than had reported 'subjective' burden (71%), as shown in Table 60.

TABLE 60

Schizophrenia
'Combined objective' burden
(by the 'subjective' burden complained of by the families)

	No or only Occasional 'Objective' Burden	*Periodic or Constant 'Objective' Burden*
No 'subjective' burden	87%	29%
Some 'subjective' burden	13%	60%
Severe 'subjective' burden		11%
All cases	19%	81%

Moreover, although 81% of these households did carry some form of 'objective' burden, only 11% of them had complained to any severe extent. On the other hand, 29% of them did not consider that they had felt any 'subjective' burden at all. There was only one case where very occasional 'objective' burden had occurred, yet some 'subjective' burden had been reported by that family.

Comparison with the total psychiatric sample (Table 39) shows that the figures were remarkably similar. The only notable difference was found in the severe 'subjective' burden group, but surprisingly the difference was in favour of the schizophrenic patients. In the total sample severe 'subjective' burden was reported in 19·6%, whereas the figure for the schizophrenic group was only 11%. At the same time, more of the families of schizophrenics denied any 'subjective' burden (29%) than did the families of the total patient group (23·6%). The differences, however, are not statistically significant.

The more favourable picture found for the schizophrenic group was none the less an interesting finding, which runs contrary to what might be expected. Their families seem to have shown greater tolerance than that found among the families of psychiatric patients in general. This unexpected degree of tolerance called for more detailed scrutiny of our data, and we tried to find out whether the degree of tolerance was equally related to the different types of 'objective' burden. We had suspected that 'subjective' burden might be greater if the patient displayed disturbing behaviour, but again this was shown not to be so; the degree of tolerance was the same irrespective of whether the 'objective' burden was due to specific adverse effects on the household or the patient's own abnormal behaviour.

We further analysed the data to see if there were any particular clusters of items or individual categories of burden which might give rise to 'subjective' burden in the family, but again we failed to find any such specific clusters; nor did the actual number of items in any one case seem to have any particular influence on the 'subjective' burden felt. Cases where six or seven items were recorded as coexisting in the one family fell as often into the 'burden' group as into the 'no burden' group.

The various adverse effects on the household, one would imagine, would be no different from what one would find in the households of non-psychiatric patients, but abnormal behaviour might well be regarded as more characteristic of psychiatric patients as such, and schizophrenic patients in particular. The fact that the 'subjective' reaction to these two different types of 'objective' burden were the same would suggest that there is not much difference subjectively for a household to have a psychiatric patient at home to care for than a physically sick one.

The discrepancy found in this group of patients between the 71% of households who subjectively felt a burden of some kind and the 81% who were objectively assessed as carrying some burden seems to provide a useful index of the tolerance extended to schizophrenics in a given community. One might perhaps more fairly draw the comparison between the 81% and only those 11% where 'subjective' burden was severe. The difference between the two aspects of the situation is then really shown in its startling extent. Where services are organized, both aspects have to be taken into account: the 'objective' burden which they aim to relieve and the 'subjective' burden felt. Neither should be taken as the sole indicator of the extent of service required. Rather the services should be so constructed that they can cater adequately for both, each in its own way.

In order to get some idea as to the relatives' attitudes to the existing services in this particular schizophrenic group, we asked them, if, looking back over the four years, they felt anything more could have been done to help either the patient or his household.

Where no 'objective' burden had occurred, naturally enough, the relatives did not feel more should have been done. Nor is it surprising that where 'objective' burden did exist, in about one-quarter (25%) of the cases, relatives felt more might well have been done. But it is remarkable that in the remaining three-quarters (75%) where some 'objective' burden existed, the relatives definitely stated that they did not think anything more could have been done. This seems to indicate a rather low level of expectation as regards therapeutic possibilities and social agency help. We show later on that in general expectation of help and similar attitudes seemed dependent more often on the 'subjective' rather than on the 'objective' burden, i.e. on how the relatives felt about the situation rather than on whether they had some actual, measurable 'objective' burden to carry.

Table 61 shows that in the case of our schizophrenic group, 8·2% of the families who did not think more could have been done complained of severe 'subjective' burden and 38% of moderate burden. The level of expectation is rather similar to what we had found for the level of the psychiatric group as a whole (see Table 45).

TABLE 61

The relatives' opinion whether more could have been done

Could more have been done?	'Subjective' Burden		
	None	Some	Severe
Yes	—	80%	20%
No	53·8%	38%	8·2%

It was difficult to find any comparable studies for our psychiatric patient group as a whole, but as regards the burden created by the schizophrenic patients some limited comparisons could be made. There are at least the three previously mentioned studies, concerning themselves with short-stay mental hospital patients (Wing *et al.*, 1964*b*), long-stay mental hospital patients (Waters *et al.*, 1965), and a group of patients largely managed in the community within a new type of mental hospital service, aimed at avoiding long-term hospitalization (Mandelbrote *et al.*, 1961 *a* and *b*). They all to some extent consider the household burden. Leyberg (1965) has also made a study of schizophrenic patients treated in a general hospital psychiatric unit similar to those under study here. He does not, however, give similar quantitative assessments of burden on the household, but descriptive accounts of the difficulties observed.

Wing *et al.* (1964*b*) only studied their sample for one year. They found that even so 43% were readmitted within that year because of disturbing behaviour, the most abnormal of which was described as being 'actively deluded', and seemed to correspond to our own category, 'odd speech and unusual ideas'. Wing *et al.* used the expression 'strained relations' in the family, which could correspond to our term 'subjective' burden; occurrence was roughly the same in Wing's and our group (59% and 60% respectively), but in our case we had nothing like his high readmission rate.

In the study by Waters *et al.* (1965) forty-two long-stay male patients were followed up for from twenty-four to fifty-two months, so the investigation was rather more comparable to ours. All the patients, however, had had to undergo an intensive rehabilitation programme before leaving the hospital. Results were better than in the previous group, and two years after discharge only 29% had been readmitted. Of the remainder, 43% showed moderate or severe disturbances in their behaviour at home, though the particular nature of it was not described. 19% caused their families severe distress, which is considerably higher than the figure of 11% severe 'subjective' burden in our group – if indeed these two items can be seen as genuinely comparable.

The impression so far gleaned is that the households of our group of schizophrenic patients on the whole felt considerably less severe 'subjective' burden than did the households of these two groups of ex-mental hospital patients. This, coupled with the high level of tolerance to 'objective' burden described above, suggests that where the chronically ill schizophrenic patient who showed disturbing behaviour and caused an amount of disruption in the home was managed largely in the community rather than in hospital *from the start* of treatment, a greater measure of acceptance was in fact created for him.

The third study (Mandelbrote *et al.*, 1961*b*) followed up a small group of schizophrenics for four years, at the end of which 69·9% were still out of hospital; 30·1% had been readmitted, were dead or could not be contacted. It is reported that 55% of the families were disturbed in some way, though it is not quite clear whether the 'burden' recorded is 'objective' or 'subjective' in our sense. Mandelbrote writes: 'typical stress situations were those in which the behaviour of the patient upset his family or prevented them from doing certain things'.

Comparable analysis is difficult as not all Mandelbrote's patients were followed up for the full four years. 16% of his patients had some or serious financial difficulties; in our group the figure for financial loss was 30%. But it must be remembered that 18% of Mandelbrote's patients stayed in hospital for the full period, and if this group is added on, we get a figure of 34%, which is much closer to ours. Similarly, although only 23% appeared moderately or severely ill in their behaviour at home compared with our figure of 60%, we have again to keep in mind that Mandelbrote's most disturbed groups (18%) were in fact in hospital and so were eliminated from these follow-up figures.

As to the 'subjective' burden, this is possibly to be paralleled with 'stress to family' in Mandelbrote's study. He reported that 2% showed severe stress, 38% some stress, while 54% appeared to have been immune. These figures are again better than ours, but the proportion of patients in hospital has once more to be kept in mind. Mandelbrote's figures, however, again illustrate the differences that exist between 'objective' and 'subjective' aspects of family burden and point along the same lines as our own study.

It would be hazardous to put too much reliance on these comparisons, but they indicate that extramural psychiatric services which hospitalize schizophrenic patients freely rather than maintain them out in the community as much as possible are likely to create less 'objective' and 'subjective' burden for the patients' families than services which steadfastly aim to reduce the hospitalization to an absolute minimum.

Attitudes to the Extramural Service The desirability of exploring attitudes in the patients and their relatives towards the new administrative arrangements has been discussed earlier (p. 110). It was shown that so far what we have called the 'tolerance' of the household towards schizophrenic patients seemed if anything to be greater than that extended towards psychiatric patients in general. Nevertheless, a certain amount of 'subjective' burden, in particular severe 'subjective' burden, did exist in the schizophrenic group and therefore the question of what the 'consumers' felt towards the service seems by no means a superfluous one to ask.

The group of patients who could be questioned on this point amounted to 45·2% of the sample. Of these 79·5% expressed satisfaction with the service and only 2·8% made any serious complaint. These latter complaints related to alleged rough handling by the nursing staff. 17·7% made what they considered to be 'minor' complaints which were very similar to what have been mentioned earlier in relation to the total psychiatric group. Such complaints cannot be directly linked to an extramural service as such, but are common to all types of hospital service, e.g. complaints of food, lack of segregation, waiting for ward rounds, etc. We have no means of comparison to establish whether our figures for complaints are high or not, in contrast with other services.

We also sought information from relatives or some constant member of the household during the four years. This was possible in 56·4% of the cases. The great majority (68·6%) said they were quite satisfied. The figure, however, is rather smaller than for the patients themselves (79·5%); similarly, the relatives had a larger number of serious complaints (8·6%). Unlike the complaints enumerated by the patients, those from the relatives seemed to have direct relevance to the effectiveness of the extramural service itself. In other words, they centred on problems which would not arise if patients were kept largely in hospital, and drew attention to what we have previously called the key factor in any extramural care – that is, adequate follow-up of the particular patient. The relatives sometimes seemed to have had a sense of 'being left alone' with the patient, and they felt acutely that there had been some breakdown in communication. A further 22·8% of the relatives had minor complaints. Here again the figure is higher than in the case of the patients, where it was 17·7%, but the nature of the complaints were similar, i.e. referring to matters common in any hospital service. It is true that in a few of these cases there was once more a feeling that greater benefit would have come from some after-care and clearer explanation of what could be expected from the patient. The relatively small number of serious complaints cannot but be reassuring to the innovators of these new psychiatric services, but one can see that there is no room for complacency and the complaints were not such as can altogether be brushed aside.

The burning question is whether the situation is similar in other types of services, but it is not yet possible to find any strictly comparable studies. Mandelbrote *et al.* (1961*a*, *b*) found in 85·4% of their cases the relatives appeared to welcome or at least accept the patient in the home, 14·6% had some reservations, and in one case there was open hostility. If one compares the figure of 85·4% with that of 68·6% in our own group – the proportion of relatives who said they were satisfied – Mandelbrote's results seem considerably better. One has to remember, however, that, as mentioned before, a large number of his group had been admitted to hospital and were kept there throughout the follow-up period (18%). Presumably therefore many of the most difficult cases had been taken off their families' hands. With our schizophrenic patients, practically the entire group lived in their community for the greater part of the four years. That households enjoy a greater sense of relief and are more satisfied with the service if the most difficult patients are screened off and admitted into hospital rather than kept under extramural care was also the finding of Grad and Sainsbury (1963). They had compared an extramural service with a conventional mental hospital service, but not so much as a follow-up study than as part of their investigation into how attitudes were affected at inception.

Wing *et al.* (1964*b*) in their study went into the question of attitudes. Theirs were short-stay patients discharged from mental hospital, who had been followed up after one year. 33% of the relatives were found to be doubtful about the patient coming home or strongly opposed, although in the event the patients had been received home. We can only surmise whether these families were satisfied or felt that something had been imposed on them. In 41% it seemed that family relations were amicable, but with the 43% of the patients who had to be readmitted, it appeared this invariably involved tension, if not distress, and, far from being satisfied, families were actively asking for the patient's removal.

These findings compare poorly with the more positive attitudes of both patients and relatives in our own schizophrenic group. It seems to suggest that if schizophrenic patients are treated on extramural lines from inception, this will engender a rather different attitude on the part of the relatives and thus tend to create a greater tolerance for the patient in the community. Considering the service was dealing with a group of patients which are thought to be particularly difficult for families to accept, the results seem remarkably satisfactory for the extramural service in this instance, nor did any of the dissatisfied informants, when questioned on this point, state that they would have preferred the patient to have been treated in the mental hospital, rather than the unit.

(II) ELDERLY PATIENTS

In the previous section we have described a diagnostically homogeneous set of patients, but the same does not apply to the elderly group which comprised all types of diagnostic categories. We studied this group separately, nevertheless, because they tend to be looked upon as a special problem in relation to the medical and social services in general. Ageing is a process which lays its mark on every clinical problem, no matter how diverse. Psychiatric patients above a certain age have greatly benefited by general attention being drawn once again to the fact that they are by no means a diagnostically homogeneous group, and that careful diagnosis must always be attempted, so as to determine the subsequent management, treatment, and prognosis (Roth and Morrissey, 1952). Nevertheless, in spite of the diversity, such patients have also a good deal in common, so that studying them together as a group becomes a useful exercise. Only recently Kay *et al.* (1966), having investigated the problem, appealed for a unification, not only of the psychiatric, but also of all the other medical and social services which deal with the problems of the old age-group.

In our case we wanted to see to what extent the elderly and aged patients in our sample engaged the services provided by the two psychiatric units – in particular, whether they made any different demands from those made by the other age-groups, and whether certain clinical and social factors affected their referral rate. In addition, we wanted to find out how this older group fared under a largely extramural type of management.

The Patients

We had a total of eighty-nine patients over sixty years of age The numbers from the two units did not differ significantly from each other and were therefore taken together. This particular age-group represented 19% of all new patients incepted by the two units in the year under survey. This is strikingly different from the situation found in other parts of the country. For instance, in another area served by a psychiatric service with an extramural orientation – namely, the Chichester area – the figures were quite different. Sainsbury and Grad (1963), who analysed this service, found that patients over sixty years comprised 37·5% of the total intake, i.e. the proportion was more than double that of our own group, a highly significant difference ($p < 0{\cdot}001$). The actual age distribution within the

TABLE 62

New inceptions by age

Age-groups, Years	Catchment Area of Burnley Unit			Catchment Area of Blackpool Unit			Catchment Areas of both Units			Catchment Area of Chichester (Sainsbury et al.)		
	Patients	%	%	Patients	%	%	Patients	%	%	Patients	%	%
14–59	369	80		412	83		781	81		443	62·5	
60–4	42	9	44·5	32	6·5	38	74	8	42·1	63	8·9	24
65–9	28	6	29·8	22	4·2	26	50	5	28·4	47	6·6	18
70 and over	24	5	25·7	30	6·3	36	54	6	29·5	155	22	58
Total	463	100	100	496	100	100	959	100	100	708	100	100

group was also very different. The patients over seventy years comprised only 29·5% of the over-sixty age-group, while a much higher proportion were between sixty and sixty-four years (42·1%). This contrasts with the Chichester findings where the percentage for the over-seventy-years group (58%) was more than double that for the sixty to sixty-four group. The difference can hardly be a chance finding ($p < 0{\cdot}01$).

In the two units under survey, the over-seventy age-group was a much smaller proportion of the clinic clientele as a whole than in Chichester. This could, of course, be due to differences in the age-distribution in the population of the catchment area itself. Chichester is known to attract a considerable number of retired people and the question naturally arises whether some such social factor is responsible for the difference in age-distribution among the patients.

Table 63, however, shows that this possibility can be safely ruled out. The figures indicate that the age-groupings in the three catchment areas of the two units on the one hand and of the Chichester Hospital on the other are very similar. The differences that do appear are not large enough to explain the marked differences in the three groups of patients.

Table 64 shows further that even if the population are broken down according to sex, the age-distribution still remains the same. It is therefore quite clear that the differences in referral rate cannot be attributed to differences in the population of the area as such. The matter is finally clinched by the figures in Table 65.

Table 65 gives the unit referral rate per 1,000 population, broken down according to sex and age. The Chichester rate for the fourteen to fifty-nine age-group was two to three times that of our two units, namely 6·37–6·41, as compared with 3·9 for the Burnley Unit and 2·5 for the Blackpool Unit. The ratio increases with increasing age, the highest difference occurring with the over-seventy female patients. In that age-group Chichester had 14·95 referrals per 1,000 population, whereas our two units had only 1·7 and 1·1 respectively. In fact the two units show a falling gradient with increasing age, while in Chichester the gradient was a rising one. This means a different usage must have taken place in these contrasted areas. In Chichester the psychiatric services were used much more

TABLE 63

Population of catchment areas

Age-groups (Years)	*Catchment Area of Blackpool Unit*		*Catchment Area of Burnley Unit*		*Catchment Area of Chichester*	
	Persons	%	*Persons*	%	*Persons*	%
14–59	164,332	70	98,247	73	69,236	73
60–9	39,349	17	20,661	15	13,404	14
70 and over	30,388	13	15,258	12	11,970	13
Total	234,069	100	134,166	100	94,610	100

TABLE 64

Population by age and sex

Age-groups	*Catchment Area of Both Units, Burnley and Blackpool*				*Catchment Area of the Chichester Service*			
	Men		*Women*		*Men*		*Women*	
60–4	13,412	33%	18,712	29%	2,839	27%	4,101	27%
65 and over	27,424	67%	46,108	71%	7,518	73%	10,958	73%
All ages over 60	40,836	100%	74,820	100%	10,357	100%	15,059	100%

TABLE 65

Referral Rates per 1,000 population
(by age and sex)

Age Groups	*Burnley Unit*		*Blackpool Unit*		*Chichester Service*	
	Men	*Women*	*Men*	*Women*	*Men*	*Women*
	3·9		2·5		6·4	
14–59	3·3	4·1	2·6	2·4		
60–4	2·9	4·3	2·1	1·1	9·16	9·02
65–9	1·6	3·9	0·8	1·4	5·42	8·65
70 and over	1·4	1·7	0·8	1·1	9·91	14·95

freely, and the higher the age-group, the more this was in evidence. The most likely reason would seem to be a different attitude in the population to the psychiatric services. The older, well-established service in Chichester enjoyed greater acceptance and was more readily used than seemed to be the case for the new services in the North, where the psychiatric units in general hospitals have only recently sprung into existence.

Another reason, however, might well be the difference in the general geriatric services in the areas investigated. Where psychiatric and general geriatric services coexist, it has been shown that admission of elderly patients to the one or the other is to a certain extent haphazard and very often inappropriate. A large number of elderly patients with predominantly psychiatric disorders are admitted to general geriatric wards, and the opposite also takes place (Kidd, 1962*b*; Kay *et al.*, 1966). That means, if external general geriatric services are available, a fair number of psychiatric patients would be channelled into these services, and thus diminish the inception rather into the psychiatric service. It is true that the two Northern catchment areas had considerable geriatric provision on which to call. For instance, in the Burnley catchment area, the total number of geriatric beds for the chronic sick amounted to 252 and in the Blackpool area to 406 beds. Furthermore, the geriatric services centred on these beds dealt with a large number of patients every year. Thus in the Burnley area the number of discharges from the geriatric beds, which gives some index of patient usage, was 486 patients per annum, and in the Blackpool area the figure was 971 patients (S.H.B., 1958 and 1959, M.O.H. publications). Unfortunately, no comparable figures are given for the Chichester area. The issue, therefore, must remain open. In order to arrive at an exact assessment of the influence the geriatric services might have on the intake of the psychiatric units, one would require some specific research. This particular investigation of ours was not designed to compass this particular question, but it has inevitably brought it to light.

It would seem that the Chichester service must have dealt largely with a different type of patient, and this difference appears in a number of aspects.

Table 66 describes the sex distribution and civil status of our patients, comparing them with the referrals at Chichester. As regards civil status, there were differences as between men and women. 70% of the men and 61% of the women were married at time of referral; 3·4% of the men and 10% of the women were single, while 26·6% of the men and 29% of the women were either widowed, separated, or divorced. When these findings are compared with those for the general population of the catchment areas, we find that the married and single men were under-represented in our sample, while the widowed, separated, and divorced were over-represented. With the women, the reverse was the case: the married were over-represented, and the single, widowed, separated, and divorced were considerably under-represented ($p < 0{\cdot}001$). The figures in the right-hand column of Table 66 illustrate once more the difference between our patients and the Chichester patients. In the latter there were much fewer married couples, and a larger number of single, widowed, and divorced persons. Although the difference is more marked in the women, it does also apply to the men.

Table 67 shows the civil status of the patients per 1,000 population. The single, widowed and divorced in Chichester had a much higher referral rate (13·43) than the married (7·86), but in our two areas the ratios of the two groups were very similar and if anything reversed. There were 1·07 single persons per 1,000 population and 1·41 married. Yet a further difference from Chichester appeared in the social-class composition of the patients.

TABLE 66

Marital state of patients and of catchment area populations
(in percentages of the total)

Sex	*Marital State*	*Burnley and Blackpool Units*		*Chichester Service*	
		Patients	*Population*	*Patients*	*Population*
Men	Married	70%	77·4%	66·9%	73%
	Single	3·4%	5·8%		
	Widowed, separated, divorced	26·6%	16·7%	34%	27%
	Total	100%	100%	100%	100%
Women	Married	61%	40·8%	28·3%	41%
	Single	10%	15·5%		
	Widowed, separated, divorced	29%	43·6%	71·7%	59%
	Total	100%	100%	100%	100%

TABLE 67

Inception rates per 1,000 population
(by marital status)
(All ages of 60 years and over)

	Burnley and Blackpool Units						*Chichester*	
	Men		*Women*		*Both Sexes*		*Both Sexes*	
	Population	*Rate per* 1000	*Population*	*Rate per* 1000	*Population*	*Rate per* 1000	*Population*	*Rate per* 1000
Married	16,432	1·26	13,925	2·58	40,357	1·41	13·733	7·86
Single	1,236	0·80	5,275	1·13	6,511	1.07	} 11,683	} 13·43
Widowed, separated, divorced	3,552	2·25	14,795	1·14	18,347	1·37		

TABLE 68

Social-class distribution amongst patients and populations (60 years and over)

		Social Class I and II	*Social Class III*	*Social Class IV and V*
Patients of units in Burnley and Blackpool	Men	26·8%	36·7%	33·5%
	Women	13·5%	54·2%	22·1%
	Both sexes	18·5%	53%	28·5%
England and Wales, aged 60 and over	Both sexes	18·3%	52·7%	29%
Chichester	Patients	42%	33%	25%
	Population aged 60 and over	24–7%	40–4%	30–4%

Table 68 shows that 18·5% of our over-sixty age-group were in the Registrar-General's Social Classes I and II, 53% in Class III, and 28·5% in Classes IV and V. Chichester had a much higher proportion in Social Classes I and II.

Our own figures correspond quite closely to the social-class distribution for England and Wales, which might lead one to conclude that social class as such did not seem to be a particularly relevant factor in referral in our catchment areas. Social Classes I and II were only very slightly over-represented in our elderly sample, and we did not find the gross over-representation of them which occurred in the Chichester services, even if we take into account that Social Classes I and II were over-represented in the Chichester area as a whole when compared with the national average.

Taking all the above differences into account, it becomes obvious that not only were the psychiatric services more used by the elderly and aged patient in the South than in the North, but social grouping also showed a different usage. Very old, single, or widowed women from Social Classes I and II, so much at risk in Chichester, were not found to any great extent among the patients in our two catchment areas. Here it was rather the married woman of from sixty to sixty-four years who was most at risk. Social class as such did not affect the issue.

In one respect our findings were not so dissimilar to those in Chichester. This was in relation to the size of the patient's household. Table 69 shows that 13·7% of our patients lived in one-person households, 54·6% shared households with one other person, and 31·7% were living in households with more than one person. These figures are more or less in line with those given by Sainsbury *et al.* (1966), who found 17% living in one-person households, 40% in two-person households, and 43% in larger households.

Sainsbury, however, could not at this time calculate the rate per 1,000 population of his catchment area in that respect. We had available the appropriate Census figures and could therefore so calculate the rate for all persons of pensionable age (i.e. all men over sixty-five, all women over sixty) in relation to the size of their household. On that basis we found a referral rate of 0·5 per 1,000 population for patients living in one-person households, 0·81 for those in two-person households, and 0·70 for those in larger households. The differences, however, were not statistically significant.

Sainsbury *et al.* suspected that patients from hotels, etc., were more frequently referred, but they emphasized that they had not enough information to make a confident statement on this point. In our sample the vast majority of our patients (89%) were either householders or lived as members of the family. Only 11% lived as lodgers in institutions or hostels. Although this proportion was small, patients living in this type of accommodation seemed over-represented in our sample as compared with the general population in the catchment area (4·3%), although we cannot be certain of this, because the Census does not report this type of living by specific age-groups. The conclusion that people living in this way are more prone to become psychiatric patients is supported by a similar finding in Chichester, where the incidence of this kind of living in the catchment area was estimated as about 4%, while among the patients it rose to 12%.

Differences from Chichester again emerge in the types of family group with whom the patients lived. Table 70 shows that in our sample 57% of the patients lived with their spouses, 19%

TABLE 69

Patients of pensionable age
(by size of households)
(Men over 65 and women over 60)

		1-Person Households	*2-Person Households*	*More than 2-Person Households*	*Total*
Units in Burnley and Blackpool	Population and inception rate per 1000	17,863 0·5	41,670 0·81	32,711 0·70	92,244 0·78
	Patients	13·7%	54·6%	31·7%	100%
Chichester	— Patients	17%	40%	43% (12% in hotels, etc.)	100%

TABLE 70

Type of household from which the patient comes
(Patients of 60 years and over)

		With Spouse	*With Grown Children*	*With Other Kin*	*Alone, Hostels, etc.*
Blackpool and Burnley units	Men	53%	20%	20%	7%
	Women	59%	18%	9%	14%
	Both sexes	57%	19%	13%	11%
Chichester	Both sexes	32%	16%	21%	31%

with their grown-up children, another 13% lived with their siblings or other kin, and 11% lived alone. In Chichester much fewer (only 32%) lived with their spouses and 31% lived either alone or in hotels, etc., as compared with 11% in our own group. Once again it is clear that psychiatric patients in the Northern areas show different sociological characteristics from psychiatric patients in the South. Diagnostic groupings are shown in Table 71. It will be seen that the majority of these

TABLE 71

Diagnoses by age

Diagnoses	*All over 60 Years*	60–4 *Years*	65–70 *Years*	70 *Years and Over*
Organic psychosyndrome	27%	17%	25%	58%
Schizophrenia	5%	—	25%	75%
Affective psychosis	49%	54%	27%	19%
Personality disorder and abnormal psychogenic reactions	14%	62%	38%	—
Other	5%	25%	25%	50%

elderly patients (49%) were suffering from affective psychoses, 27% had organic psychosyndromes, 14% showed personality disorders and abnormal psychogenic reactions, 5% were schizophrenics (all of them women), and 5% had other diagnoses. Compared with the findings in Chichester, our group seemed to have fewer organic psychosyndromes – namely, as compared with 47·2% in Chichester ($p < 0·01$) – possibly because we had a smaller number of patients over seventy years of age. As regards the other diagnostic categories, the descriptions unfortunately are not comparable. Table 71 shows how the diagnostic categories in our sample distributed themselves over the three different sub-groups. It can be seen that, whereas the affective psychoses (54%) and the personality disorders (62%) were more frequently found in the two lower age-groups, the organic psychosyndromes (58%) were more frequent in the upper age-group. The schizophrenics were too few to be the subject of comment.

Many of our patients, although incepted at the units for the first time, had been ill for a considerable period previously, just as in the Chichester group. In fact, 37% had been so for over two years, and another 34% for periods ranging from six months to two years. Only 29% had been ill for less than six months at the time of inception. More of our group had been ill for the longer time than was the case with the elderly patients in Chichester (37% of our patients, as contrasted with 30% of the Chichester patients), and as many as 55% had been ill for less than six months in Chichester, compared with our 29%. Perhaps these figures lend support to the view that there is some greater reluctance in the North to use the psychiatric services, and this leads to some postponement in referral. Table 72 also shows the larger proportion of chronic sick in the aged group (over seventy years of age). The figure here is 42%, while that for the short-term illnesses is only 16%. In the sixty to sixty-four age-group, however, the proportions are reversed (28% as compared with 46%).

Conclusions

It seems, then, on looking back over the above findings, that the upper age-groups in the population do not make any unduly high demand on a psychiatric service such as is described here. The demand was in fact lower than that of the younger age-groups (under sixty years). Moreover, the older patients appeared to form only a relatively small percentage of

TABLE 72

Duration of illness before inception
(by age-groups)
(60 years and over)

Duration of Illness	*Chichester*	*Blackpool and Burnley Units*	*Blackpool and Burnley Units*		
			60–4	65–9	*70 and over*
Up to 6 months	55%	29%	46%	38%	16%
7–24 months	15%	34%	53%	17%	30%
Over 2 years	30%	37%	28%	30%	42%

the entire clientele of the units. Less than two out of ten new inceptions would be in that age-group. The Chichester findings led us to expect rather different results. Though it was a type of service in some ways very similar to the one studied here, it was used generally to a much greater extent, and even more so by the older group of patients. There the older age-group seemed to be a major and growing burden on the comprehensive service, whereas in these Northern areas so far this did not seem to be the case.

This difference in usage may well be due to different attitudes to the psychiatric service amongst the populations concerned. Historical reasons probably entered, since the psychiatric units in the North had been in existence for a much shorter length of time than those in the South. In the North they were not so well known, and there seemed a greater reluctance to use them, which seems confirmed by the longer duration of the psychiatric illness before referral to the unit came at last.

Management of the Elderly Patient

Use of In-patient Services

Our main object in investigating the elderly group of psychiatric patients was to see to what extent they required hospitalization, or more precisely to what extent the policy of the psychiatric unit of avoiding long-term hospitalization was achieved in their case. Since the elderly tend to suffer more from progressive or at least irreversible diseases and since mental illness is very frequently accompanied by non-psychiatric disorder, it is not unnatural to suspect that unit policy might founder, or at least not succeed to the same extent as it did with its younger patients.

In fact, we found that, even amongst the elderly, the patients were in general very little hospitalized over the four years. 17% had never been in-patients at all, not even at inception; another 66% had not stayed in hospital for more than three months throughout the period; 11% had spent a total of from four to twelve months in hospital, and only 6% had spent one year and over. The figures (Table 23) represent the aggregate hospital time (unit and/or mental hospital), over the four

TABLE 73

Aggregate in-patient stay in mental hospital
(Patients of 60 years and over)

Aggregate In-patient Stay in Mental Hospital	*Blackpool and Burnley Units*				*Chichester, All Patients over 60*
	Total Age-groups over 60	*60–4 Years*	*65–9 Years*	*70 Years and Over*	
Never	88·6%	94%	88%	81·5%	39%
Up to 3 months	4·5%	3%	8%	3·7%	61% (combined)
4–12 months	1·2%	3%	—	—	
1 year and over	5·6%	—	4%	14·8%	

years, and comparison may be made with the under-sixty age-group.

It can be seen that as far as long-stay hospitalization is concerned, the elderly patient can be managed in the same way as the rest of the psychiatric group. The only significant difference arose among patients who had no admissions at all. The figures here are 17% for the elderly, in contrast to 33% for the younger group. The difference is made up by the short-term admissions, which were more frequent for the older age-group, and appeared to occur, almost exclusively, immediately upon inception at the unit. In other words, about one-third of the younger age-group were treated as out-patients or day-patients after being first seen at the unit, while a larger number of the elderly group were admitted as in-patients at this point, but they stayed less than three months in all. It was not possible to elicit the actual difference in detail, but it seems plausible to suppose that physical conditions in the elderly group were predominantly responsible for this kind of management.

The figures so far mentioned refer to the 'total hospital time', irrespective of whether this was spent in the units or the mental hospitals. They seem impressive enough. However, when the 'total hospital time' is divided up according to whether the time was spent in the unit or in the mental hospital, we find that the mental hospital service was indeed very little used. As many as 88·6% of the elderly patients never were in mental hospital, and of the 11·4% remaining, nearly half (4·5%) only stayed from three to twelve months and only 5·6% spent a total time of over one year. With such findings as these, we can hardly talk about large-scale, long-term mental hospital stay at all.

Table 73 shows how little the mental hospital service was in fact used, both as regards the number referred to it and the length of time spent by each patient.

Hospitalization in the units, on the other hand, presented quite a different picture. Here it was the majority of the patients – namely, 81% – who were admitted as in-patients, but the situation was still similar to that prevailing in the mental hospital service when this came to the length of time the patient spent in the unit. The largest group (40%) had a 'total hospital time' of less than one month. The total picture emerging from these figures is that of a generous use made by the units of very brief in-patient admissions, these falling mainly in the inception period rather than during the subsequent four years.

TABLE 74

Aggregate in-patient stay in unit
(Patients of 60 years and over)

Aggregate In-patient Stay in Unit	*Both Units*			
	Total	60–4 *Years*	65–9 *Years*	70 *Years and Over*
Never	19%	22%	16%	19%
1–4 weeks	40% } 81%	44%	44%	32%
5–12 weeks	29% } 81%	27%	32%	30%
13 weeks and over	12% } 81%	7%	8%	19%

Table 74 shows that increasing age did not appear to affect in-patient admission rates to any great extent, so far as the units were concerned, although the longer-term patients (staying four months or more) did show a higher proportion of the seventy age-group and over. We find 19% in that group, as contrasted with 7–8% in the under-seventies.

In the case of in-patient admission to the mental hospital, the difference becomes more marked. 14·8% of the seventy and over age-group are found to be longer-stay patients, as compared with only 4% of the sixty-five to sixty-nine age-group, and none at all in the sixty to sixty-four age-group. Thus the

TABLE 75

Aggregate morbidity during the follow-up period
(by age-groups)
(60 years and over)

Aggregate Duration of Illness	*Total*	60–4 *Years*	65–9 *Years*	70 *Years and Over*
1–6 months	20%	42%	42%	16%
7–24 months	26%	50%	19%	31%
Over 2 years	54%	30%	30%	40%

aged patients used in-patient facilities more, and this becomes particularly noticeable in respect to the mental hospital usage.

Morbidity

As we have shown above, this group of elderly and aged patients had been ill for a considerable time before inception. It will therefore not come as a surprise to find that a good deal of morbidity existed during the follow-up period as well. Table 75 gives an idea of the extent of this morbidity. It shows that 54% were ill for more than half the follow-up period, 26% were ill for periods of from seven to twenty-four months, while in only 20% was the aggregate morbidity less than six months. As might be expected, the aged – those over seventy years – did worse, although the difference with the other age-groups was not very marked. 40% were ill for more than two years and only 16% for less than six months, whereas in the sixty to sixty-four age-group, 42% had been ill for less than six months and 30% for more than two years.

Concomitant Non-psychiatric Illness

The presence of mental disorder does by no means preclude the presence of other physical illnesses, and this applies particularly to the upper age-groups. In geriatric practice, single pathologies are the exception, and good medical practice must address itself to the whole patient and the complexity of his situation. To what extent this is achieved will be a measure of the care given, particularly where there are elderly patients. We therefore tried to assess the extent of non-psychiatric illness in our patient group and how it was affected by the extramural management.

For this purpose we did not include patients who were referred to the units because of an organic psychosyndrome, although gross organic illness might be present, e.g. cerebral arteriosclerosis. We only included those conditions which were present in addition to the pathology giving rise to the psychosyndrome.

A fairly large proportion (33%) had such additional non-psychiatric illness at the time of inception. This proportion was the same for all the age-groups over sixty years. Another 15% of the patients fell ill with major non-psychiatric disorders subsequent to inception. That meant that nearly half of the patients were suffering some gross physical disability in addition to any organic psychosyndrome that might be present.

The aggregate duration of the physical ill-health during the follow-up period was quite extensive. Of the forty-four patients on whom accurate information was available 57% were physically ill for at least two years, 28% were ill for from one to two years, and 15% were ill for less than six months. Men and women were affected to the same extent and the specific age-groupings showed no difference either. It can thus be seen that the over-sixty age-group were a chronically ill population for the most part, and a considerable number remained ill for long periods during the follow-up time, even after inception, both mentally and physically.

Mortality

Finally, as might be expected, a high percentage of our group (39%) died during the follow-up period, as shown in Table 76.

TABLE 76

Mortality
(by age-groups)
(60 years and over)

	Total	60–4 *Years*	65–9 *Years*	70 *Years and Over*
Died	39%	31%	26%	43%
Alive	61%	48%	30%	22%

The proportions for men and women proved similar, but naturally there was a higher death-rate among the aged group (over seventy years). The figure here is 43% ($p < 0{\cdot}01$). How these figures compare with those found in the general population of the catchment area is described and discussed in Section III (p. 193ff.). They were in fact higher than in the general population, which is not surprising, although not as high as the figures quoted for mental hospital populations. No patient died of suicide, and in most cases death was due to vascular disease, malignancy, respiratory disease, and so on. Again these findings are discussed in more detail in Section III.

Use of Other Services

Since this patient group was so ill and yet spent so little time in hospital, one may wonder to what extent the burden of their care devolved on other medical and social services.

General Practitioner

Contact with the general practitioner was much more frequent among the over-sixty age-group than among the sample as a whole: 61% of the older age-group and 35% of the total sample had frequent or regular contacts (i.e. about once a month on average). The difference is highly significant ($p < 0{\cdot}001$). The total sample was already using general practitioner services in excess of the general population, as was shown earlier (see p. 87). We do not know the rate of usage of general practitioners for non-psychiatric over-sixty age-groups, but it seems likely that in this case also the psychiatric group would use the general practitioner more frequently. In our particular inquiry we had no means of ascertaining whether the consultations with the general practitioner were for psychiatric reasons or other reasons or both. Men patients tended to use their general practitioner more frequently than the women patients, but the difference was not significant.

In general, therefore, our group of elderly, chronically sick psychiatric patients, many of whom had non-psychiatric illnesses as well, did not put an excessive burden on the general practitioner services, though it seems that they required rather more attention than the general population at large.

Domiciliary Visits

54% of the group were incepted by domiciliary visits, slightly more than in the case of our total sample (37%), but both these figures are much higher than that quoted for comparable patients by Kessel (1965) in his Plymouth study, where only 11% of the elderly were domiciliary patients on inception. However, similar trends were observed in both studies, i.e. the older the patients the more often domiciliary visits were made. For instance, in our sample in the sixty to sixty-four age-group 40% were domiciliary inceptions, in the sixty-five to sixty-nine age-group 50% of the patients were so incepted, and the figure for the seventy years and over age-group was 63%. As in Plymouth, more women (59%) received domiciliary visiting than men (44%), but the difference in our group was not so marked as in Plymouth.

After this fairly lavish use of domiciliary visiting at inception, this service was little called upon thereafter. Only some 3% of the patients had more than one initial domiciliary visit, and there was no difference in this follow-up pattern between the elderly patients and the younger age-groups. Over the four years, therefore, there was no substantial demand for continued domiciliary care.

Since the Plymouth service was essentially based on the mental hospital, the difference in domiciliary visiting would suggest that the general hospital psychiatric unit tends to work closer to the community, whereas the Plymouth service, waiting for the patients to come forward rather than attending to them in their homes, tended to be more hospital-centred. Although the centre investigated by Kessel represented an attempt to come closer to the community, the general hospital psychiatric unit, nevertheless, seems to have achieved this to a greater extent.

Other Psychiatric Unit Services (Non-in-patient)

Only 14% of our elderly group had been incepted as out-patients – a very much lower percentage than that found in the Plymouth study, but not too far out of step with the distribution of the other age-groups in our total sample. During the subsequent four years 56% made use of these services to the extent of from one to ten attendances, 6% attended from eleven to twenty-four times, and only 3% attended twenty-five times or more. 35% of the patients did not attend at all during the four years. The day-hospital facilities, which were only beginning to develop, had an equally light usage. Only 9% of the elderly patients used these facilities, 5% for an aggregate duration of six months over the four years and another 4% for a period of from one to two years. Neither sex nor increasing age appeared to have any determining influence. It would seem, therefore, that it cannot be said that this group of elderly psychiatric patients created any substantial load on the out-patient or day-patient facilities, and indeed used them rather less than the total sample as a whole.

General Hospital In-patient Admissions

Kidd (1962) has shown that psychiatric geriatric patients often drift into general hospital beds. However, in our sample only 6% of these elderly patients were in a general hospital for more than an aggregate of twelve weeks throughout the four years. If this was due to 'wrong hospitalization' in the sense in which Kidd uses the phrase, the percentage is very small. The large majority of our patients (67%) were never general hospital in-patients at all. The remaining 27% stayed less than an aggregate of twelve weeks in the four years and of these as many as 18% stayed less than four weeks. It would seem that these short-term admissions must have been for straightforward medical purposes and were not covert methods of psychiatric disposal. No difference in usage was found as between the sexes. It will be seen, therefore, that a total of 33% of our elderly group did make use of general hospital in-patient facilities, but the majority of them only for very short-term stays. Thus they made a larger use of the hospital than did the younger age-group, where this figure was only 21%, but the difference is not significant.

General Hospital Out-patient Service

Absolute numbers here are small and comment can only be guarded. The general hospital out-patient services were attended by 18% of the men (15% for from one to five attendances, 3% for from six to twelve attendances). More of the men patients belonged to the aged (over-seventy years) group. The average attendance at general hospital out-patients of non-psychiatric elderly and aged patients is not known, but it is likely that our group had a more frequent attendance rate, though it does not seem a very high one over the four years, and was indeed smaller than that for the psychiatric sample as a whole.

Social Agencies

The supporting social services were used by 37% of our over-sixty age-group and there was little difference between the sexes as to the amount of usage. Nor was there any age gradient. It is interesting that the usage was not so very different from that of our total psychiatric sample, where 39% had received some social agency care throughout the four years, this figure being to some extent swelled by the usage of the Ministry of Labour in the case of the younger group of employable patients. For a more detailed analysis of the usage of the social services, we would refer the reader to pp. 92ff.

Conclusions

The above findings seem to confirm that the patients in the over-sixty age-groups as well as those in the under-sixty groups could both be managed in an extramural psychiatric service without putting an undue burden on the supporting out-patient and domiciliary services of the units or on the general hospital, general practitioner, or social services. This was so, despite the fact that this geriatric group carried a good deal of non-psychiatric chronic ill-health as well as chronic psychiatric illness throughout the four years under survey. It is true the older psychiatric patients appeared to engage the general practitioner rather more than non-psychiatric patients tend to do so, but one could not say the claim was at all excessive, and the burden devolved on the general practitioner could hardly be called overwhelming.

The next question which naturally arises from the foregoing is whether the relatively slight support from out-patient, day-patient, or social agency services meant that the patients' families had been left to cope with unduly difficult situations.

Effects on the Household

The elderly psychiatric patient can be expected to create certain serious difficulties; often he lives alone or shares his home with another elderly, infirm person, who may also suffer from some chronic debilitating illness. Furthermore, as a group they may be expected to need a good deal of care and attention from their relatives, who may be hard pressed with other domestic calls.

Using the method of assessing 'burden' as described above (pp. 97-8), we first assessed the 'objective' burden created by our elderly group in terms of adverse effects on the household.

TABLE 77

'Objective' burden
Adverse effects on household
(Patients of 60 years and over)

Type of 'Objective' Burden caused by Patient's Illness	*Households affected*
Financial:	
Financial status of patient or of household has suffered	7%
Any member of household has lost earnings	9%
Any member of household had to start going out to work	1%
Health:	
Physical strain caused by patient's illness to any member of the household	some, 11%; marked, 5% } 16%
Poor health in any member of the household	3%
Children:	
Separation of children under 16 from their parents	not applicable
Distress in children under 16	not applicable
General:	
Disruption of the life of any member of the household	some, 23%; much, 21% } 44%
Any kind of objective adverse effect (N = 61)	66%

Table 77 shows that the different items which constitute this type of burden. The highest figure (44%) was in the category of 'disruption of family routine', but effects were only serious in 21%. Physical strain occurred in 16% of the families, causing actual illness in another 3%. Financial loss was not great, as might be expected in this group, since only the sixty-to-sixty-five-year-old patients could be expected to be wage-earners. In 9% other members of the household lost earnings, possibly because they had to stay at home to look after the patient. In 7% either patient or household had suffered a loss of income, which in 1% of the families had had the effect of making another household member take up work to supplement income. As we were dealing with an elderly population, there were scarcely any young children under sixteen years, and separation from parents did not arise.

There was, of course, a certain amount of overlap in the individual burdens and several adverse effects could coincide in *any* one household. When all households were counted in which *any* adverse effect had been operative, it was found that 66% were so affected as a result of the patient's illness. If the figure seems high at first glance, it must be remembered that not only constant but periodic effects were included here, and these latter need not have been very frequent during the four-year period.

Generally speaking, this type of 'objective' burden was found to be related to the fact that so many of these patients were organically ill. The older age-group caused more physical strain on their families through the need for nursing care than did the younger age-group, though they were less of a charge in respect to financial loss or the separation of young children from home. It is interesting that at least 34% of the elderly patients appeared to create no such burden for their families at all.

Table 78 lists the various kinds of abnormal behaviour thought to be distressing to relatives and reported by them as occurring constantly or periodically during the four-year period. Item 9 – behaviour needing physical or nursing care – shows the highest percentage of families affected (27%), which is no doubt connected with the high incidence of terminal illness in the patient group. Item 10 – excessive demand for companionship – showed the next highest incidence (21%); this is followed by apparent wilful unco-operativeness (Item 6) and other unusual behaviour (Item 11), each affecting 20% of the families. The latter item includes a variety of behaviour not otherwise covered – namely, (1) hostile, irritable behaviour,

TABLE 78

'Objective' burden
disturbing behaviour
(Patients of 60 years and over)

Type of Disturbing Behaviour	*Burden*	
	Constant or Periodic	*Occasional*
1. Noisy or wandering at night	17%	1%
2. Dangerous to themselves or to others	17%	7%
3. Unacceptable sexual behaviour	2%	—
4. Generally restless, noisy, or talkative	6%	1%
5. Unresponsive	8%	—
6. Apparently wilfully unco-operative	20%	1%
7. Used odd speech or expressed 'unusual ideas'	18%	1%
8. Hypochondriasis	11%	—
9. Requiring nursing or physical care	27%	3%
10. Demanding excessive companionship	21%	—
11. Other unusual behaviour	20%	2%
Any type of disturbing behaviour (N = 58)	72%	28%

(2) behaviour calling for watchfulness, (3) offensive personal habits, (4) extreme seclusiveness. The next highest incidence was found under Items 1, 2, and 7 – namely, noisy and wandering at night (17%), dangerous to self and others (17%), and using odd speech or expressing unusual ideas (18%). Hypochondriasis was found to a slightly less extent (11%) and so was general unresponsiveness (8%). Restlessness and talkativeness were found in 6% and unacceptable sexual behaviour in 2%.

If we take all types of disturbing behaviour together, we find that 72% of our group displayed some type of constant or periodic disturbing behaviour which might be thought to constitute some burden for their households. These results again reflect the fact that the psychiatric units were dealing with a group of patients who for the most part were physically ill as well as mentally, in that this older age-group showed a higher incidence in almost every item compared with the sample as a whole, but the most striking difference appears in the items linked with physical ill-health, e.g. nursing care and the call for excessive companionship and attention. Even so 28% showed no disturbing behaviour at all or did so only very occasionally during the four years.

The two types of burden seem very different in nature, yet they occurred in fact to a very similar extent. They differed only in that disturbing behaviour appeared more marked in the over-sixty-five age-group, whereas adverse effects on the household seemed equally present throughout all the over-sixty age-groups. There also seemed to be a higher degree of family tolerance towards the disturbing behaviour than towards the other type of burden. In the latter case only 2·7% of the families had no subjective complaint to make, whereas this figure rose to 13% in the case of the former.

Combined 'Objective' Burden It was found that only one-fifth (20%) of the patients had managed to create no type of 'objective' burden of any kind for their family. The vast majority (80%) did pose some problem or other, and there was a trend for this burden to increase with increasing age, though differences were not significant. It will be appreciated that the figures do not take into account whether patients created more than one difficulty, nor whether this was constant or periodic, but very occasional difficulties were not counted as burden.

Table 79 shows that diagnosis was an important factor. If the group is divided into those patients who created burden and those who did not, we find that the organic psychosyndromes tended to fall into the 'burden' group (34%) rather than into the 'no burden' group (22%). Affective psychoses, on the other hand, showed a reverse trend. It is interesting that schizophrenics as well as patients with personality disorders and abnormal psychogenic reactions were equally represented in the 'burden' and 'no burden' groups.

TABLE 79

'Combined objective' burden
(by diagnosis)
(Patients of 60 years and over)

	Organic Psychosyndrome	*Schizophrenia*	*Affective Psychosis*	*Personality Disorder and Abnormal Psychogenic Reaction*	*Other*
No burden	22%	5%	56%	13%	4%
Burden	34%	4%	44%	14%	4%

Table 80 shows that the aggregate duration of psychiatric morbidity correlated significantly with whether the patient appeared in the 'burden' or 'no burden' group ($p < 0{\cdot}02$). The longer the psychiatric illness lasted, the more likely the patient fell into the 'burden' group. As regards non-psychiatric ill-health, however, there was no such relationship unless the illness was terminal; the proportion of the dead in the 'burden' group amounted to 6%.

TABLE 80

'Combined objective' burden
(by aggregate duration of mental and physical ill-health)
(Patients 60 years and over)

	Aggregate Duration of Ill-health	*Less than One Month*	*1–24 Months*	*2 Years and Over*
No	Mental	60%	28%	12%
Burden	Physical	60%	15%	25%
Burden	Mental	8%	34%	58%
	Physical	43%	26%	31%

The aggregate length of stay in the unit as an in-patient did not affect the issue, but a larger number of those who had been in mental hospital were in the 'burden' group – namely, 15·8%

as compared with 5% in the 'no burden' group. But it did not seem to matter very much how long they had stayed in the mental hospital.

TABLE 81

'Combined objective' burden
(social agency care given)
(Patients of 60 years and over)

	Social Agency Care given			
	None	*Occasional*	*Periodic*	*Constant*
No burden	78%	9%	4%	9%
Burden	51%	29%	6%	14%

Table 81 further shows that the amount of social agency care differed for the 'burden' and 'no burden' group. Periodic or constant social care was given to 20% in the 'burden' group and 13% in the 'no burden' group. The figures for occasional care were 29% and 9% respectively, while 51% in the 'burden' group and 78% in the 'no burden' group received no social care at all. It would seem that to some extent social care was properly directed towards the families that carried some 'objective' burden, but there remained a fairly large group where, although 'objective' burden was present, no social care had been received.

Although the combined 'objective' burden appeared considerable, the 'subjective' burden, as reported by relatives, did not entirely coincide with it. In 29% of those cases where there had been 'objective' burden complaints from the relatives were severe, in 57% the complaints were moderate, and in 14% there had been no 'subjective' complaints at all. This last figure (14%) is in some sense a measure of the tolerance in the community of psychiatric illness in the elderly. Compared with the figures for the total psychiatric sample, there is clearly less tolerance for the older patient (see p. 111). In the total sample only 19·6% had complained of severe 'subjective' burden, although 'objective' burden was being carried, and as many as 23·6% had no complaint to make at all. However, when relatives were asked if they felt more could have been done to help the patient or the family, only very few (6%) felt that this was so. These were all households which were carrying some 'objective' burden. In view therefore of the relatively high incidence of 'subjective' burden this last finding would suggest a very low expectation in the households of these elderly patients regarding the help that the medical and social services might provide.

'Subjective' Burden It was seen above that 'subjective' burden (i.e. what the relatives themselves felt and to what extent they considered the patient's illness had been a burden to them) did not coincide wholly with the amount of 'objective' burden carried. We therefore examined various clinical and social factors which might have influenced the relatives' attitudes as such, irrespective of whether any 'objective' burden was being carried or not. We found that 38% of the households had not complained of any 'subjective' burden at all over the four years; another 41% had complained of slight or moderate burden and 21% had complained of severe burden. Thus the 'burden' is higher than for the total psychiatric sample (see p. 105), and would again suggest that the elderly psychiatric patient is not so well tolerated in the home.

The factors of age, sex, marital status, and social class played no part at all. The organic psychosyndromes were the only diagnostic group that showed any significant difference. They were represented in the 'no burden' group with only 18%, but with 39% in the 'some or severe burden' group. The difference was of borderline significance ($p\ 0{\cdot}05$). The other diagnostic groups were represented equally in both the 'burden' and 'no burden' groups. Duration of mental ill-health, as shown in Table 82, did have a marked effect.

Of the relatives of those whose illness lasted under one month, only 5% complained of 'subjective' burden, whereas 65% did not. But when the illness had lasted over two years, the difference was markedly reversed, 55% complained of 'subjective' burden, while 13% did not ($p < 0{\cdot}001$). It is interesting to see that the duration of non-psychiatric illnesses did not show any significant relationship. Terminal illness and death, however, were highly significant. Only 13% in the 'no burden'

TABLE 82

'Subjective' burden
(aggregate duration of mental or physical ill-health)
(Patients of 60 years and over)

	Aggregate Duration of Ill-health	*Less than 1 Month*	*1–24 Months*	*2 Years and Over*
No 'subjective' burden	Mental	65%	22%	13%
	Physical	87%	13%	30%
Some or severe 'subjective' burden	Mental	5%	40%	55%
	Physical	42%	26%	29%

group had died during the follow-up period, whereas of those where 'subjective' burden had arisen, 65% had died ($p < 0{\cdot}001$).

Whether patients had been unit in-patients was not a factor significantly relevant to 'subjective' burden, but all those who had been in mental hospital were in the 'burden' group (13%). That is, mental hospitalization did not occur unless there was 'subjective' burden, which presumably exerted pressure for the patient's removal. But 'subjective' burden did by no means always have this effect, since the majority of cases (87%), where relatives complained of 'subjective' burden never went to mental hospital at all. Although there was this slight connection between 'subjective' burden and admission to mental hospital, how long the patient stayed there was not determined by the 'subjective' burden on the household. The two did not correlate.

Social care was to a certain extent directed towards the families who complained of 'subjective' burden. Whereas in the 'no burden' group only 2·6% received social care, in the 'burden' group the figure was enlarged to 53%. The difference is significant ($p < 0{\cdot}02$). 7% of the households complained that more might have been done. They were in the 'burden' group. This is substantially less than the amount of 'subjective' burden complained of, so that expectancy of service was low.

Conclusions

There are no reports in the literature which would enable us to make accurate comparisons. The closest is the report by Sainsbury and Grad (1963). They recorded similar types of burden, but they made a point prevalence assessment at time of referral, whereas we assessed a four-year prevalence. Furthermore, they investigated only those patients who were over sixty-five years, and in presenting their figures gave only the percentage of those where 'burden' had applied, taking this as a percentage of a varied total after exclusion of the 'not known'. Thus our figures would have to be modified somewhat to make them comparable. But, bearing these points in mind, their findings are remarkably similar in that they also had a high incidence of 'burden' caused by nursing care and the need of the patient for excessive companionship.

In our sample, tolerance of relatives towards 'objective' burden was present. Although this figure seems rather low, as we have seen, hardly any relatives felt that more could have been done, indicating a low expectancy as to the degree to which medical and social services could help to relieve burden. There was no difference here between the older age-groups and the total sample. Such a low expectancy would, of course, if shared by those responsible for organizing services, amount to complacency. As extramural types of care expand, there is a clear need for further research, so that available resources can be more effectively turned to examine such problems.

As regards 'subjective' burden as such, we found more relatives complained in the case of the elderly group of patients than with the total sample. Severe complaints formed 21% in the elderly group as compared with 13·9% for all age-groups. Subjective burden was also mostly related to non-psychiatric ill-health in the same way as the 'objective' burden, i.e. it was highest with the organic psychosyndromes of long duration or when terminal illness had occurred. Admission of the elderly patients to the unit in no way correlated with the relatives' subjective complaints, i.e. decision to admit to the unit was made mainly on clinical grounds, irrespective of the pressure of complaint. With mental hospital admissions, however, the relatives' 'subjective' burden did seem to play a certain part.

No patient went to mental hospital who came from a family where there was no 'subjective' burden. It is true that those who went to mental hospital were only a minority of the patients who caused 'subjective' burden to their families, but it would seem that this burden was at least one of the factors that exerted pressure in that direction.

It appears, therefore, that elderly psychiatric patients do present a greater problem if managed in an extramural type of service than the younger age-groups. They tend to create a greater amount of 'objective' burden for their households and the households themselves are more sensitive to the burden and less willing to bear it. Nevertheless, 'subjective' complaints in relation to the elderly in this investigation did not amount to any pressure to have the patients hospitalized in every case, nor in fact did these patients make greater demands on most of the services than the psychiatric sample as a whole.

(III) MORTALITY

The mortality amongst psychiatric patients has received some attention, in particular in relation to psychiatric services. All studies agree that mental hospital patients show a higher death-rate than the general population (Malzberg, 1934; Shepherd, 1957; Norris, 1959). The causes for this are complex and may be partly related to factors inherent in psychiatric illness, but may also be related to the service itself. All this makes it pertinent to ask whether the death-rate amongst patients cared for by an extramural type of psychiatric service, such as we have investigated here, is any different from that amongst patients in a conventional mental hospital service.

Change in either direction could be expected. It might be argued that in an extramural psychiatric service so closely linked to a general hospital the level of general medical care for the patients might be higher and consultation with other specialists could be arranged with a greater facility, while the ancillary services for investigation and treatment of non-psychiatric illness could be more readily available. Thus one might expect that patients in such a service would show a lower death-rate than those in a mental hospital service. In addition one might argue that admission to mental hospital and prolonged stay in such an institution could of itself be traumatic in many cases, particularly in the older age-group, and might be one of the factors that hasten death.

On the other hand, it is also arguable to the contrary that patients in an extramural service may be more at risk if left much of the time with their relatives rather than being in the care of trained nurses and doctors in the mental hospital. According to this argument, patients who spend most of the time out of hospital become exposed more grossly to the effects of serious illness, and thus may well show an overall higher death-rate than mental hospital patients. We addressed ourselves to this very problem and found the situation with our own sample to be as follows:

The Patients

There were in all fifty-four patients who died during the four years. There were twenty-three men (42%) and thirty-one women (58%). Of the fifty-four patients, sixteen (30%) were less than sixty years of age and thirty-eight patients (70%) were over sixty years. Twenty-three patients (43%) had died in the first year of follow-up, but quite a large proportion – namely, 9% of the total – had died in the first month after inception and another 17% during the first six months. Eight patients (15%) had died within the second year and fifteen patients (28%) within the third year. The final and fourth year accounted for five patients (9%), while for the remaining three patients (5%) the precise date of death could not be established.

Comparisons with Mental Hospital

The question of whether the death-rate in our patient group was higher than in the mental hospital services could not be answered satisfactorily. Such statistics as exist, or at least such as we could find, merely analyse the death-rate amongst the in-patient admissions to mental hospital. In most mental hospital services psychiatrists are reluctant to admit patients who present with mild forms of illness, and take in only those whose illness is too severe for the patient to remain as an outpatient. Because of this selection, mental hospital in-patient statistics deal with a much more severely ill group of people than those contained in our own sample, which included all types of psychiatric patient, many of whom would have remained as out-patients in an ordinary mental hospital service. Thus the patients in our total sample were not strictly comparable with those in the mental hospital statistics, and this limited comparability must be borne in mind when evaluating the subsequent data.

Column III in Table 83 shows the death-rate among the in-patients in London mental hospitals who had been admitted between 1947 and 1949 (Norris, 1959). The figures represent the death-rate within the first year of admission. It will be noted that the age-groupings used by Norris are somewhat different from our own, and therefore are not strictly comparable. Nevertheless, it is quite obvious that her figures are not only grossly in excess of those found in the general population (given in column II), but also of the figures for the death-rate in our own sample (given in column I). In fact, her figures are from two to three times as high as ours.

Another study of the death-rate among first admissions to a county mental hospital was reported by Shepherd (1957). His findings seem to repeat the same trend as Norris's. The figures are given in column IV. Shepherd studied two groups of first admissions to his county mental hospital. The first group was admitted between 1931 and 1933 and the second group between 1945 and 1948. The burden of Shepherd's findings was that the patients admitted in the latter triennium had already the benefit of the post-war developments in psychiatric administrative reform and therapeutics, and showed a shorter average stay in hospital than those of the pre-war triennium. His figures as regards the death-rate show that the sixteen to sixty-four age-groups had a much lower death-rate after the war than before. Pre-war the rate was 212 per 1,000 population, and this had fallen to 116 in the post-war triennium. Among the older patients (sixty-five years and over) there had also been a fall, but only a slight one, from 667 to 647 per 1,000 population. Thus not even the new, open-door policy of 1945–8, which had become well established in that particular hospital, had brought the death-rate down to the level observable among our own sample of patients in an extramural service. In our sample the

TABLE 83

Death-rates per 1,000 population
(According to age-groups)

I		II		III		IV	
New Admissions to units in Blackpool and Burnley within the first year after inception		*General Population of England and Wales*		*Mental Hospital In-patient Admissions in 1947–9 within First Year after Admission (V. Norris)*		*New Admissions to a County Mental Hospital within the First Year after Admission (Shepherd)*	
						1931–3	1945–8
65 years and over	230·7	85 years and over	223·2	Men, 65 years and over	821·1	65 years and over 667	647
		75–84 years	99·2	Women	385·5		
		65–74 years	39·9				
60–4 years	135	55–64 years	15·9	Men, 45–64 years	273·7		
				Women	130·7	16–64 years 212	116
16–59 years	16·6	16–54 years	0·65–15·9	Men, 16–44 years	36·6		
				Women	37		

sixteen to fifty-nine age-groups had a death-rate of 16·6 per 1,000 population; the sixty to sixty-four age-group showed a much higher rate of 135 per 1,000 population, but even the sixty-five years and over age-group only showed a rate of 230·7 per 1,000 population. This difference between the death-rate of our own patients and those found by Norris and Shepherd are all the more striking if one takes into account the fact that their figures included only those deaths that occurred while patients were actually in hospital, and disregarded those that occurred at home or elsewhere, though originally the patients might have been in-patients and under observation at some time within the years under survey. The entire patient intake therefore was by no means accounted for. We, on the other hand, treated our intake of new patients at the units strictly as one cohort, and followed each patient up irrespective of whether they died in hospital or not, and so included all the deaths.

Thus the death-rates given by Norris and Shepherd are almost certainly an underestimate in the context of this comparison. We can therefore state confidently that the death-rate amongst first admissions in an extramural psychiatric service is considerably lower than that among first admissions to the conventional mental hospital services.

In order to enable comparison with other investigations, we have so far had to use the death-rate *during the first year after inception* only. It seemed possible, however, that an extramural type of service might show up to disadvantage by curtailing longevity only when the long-term effect of its management was considered. It seemed of interest, therefore, to examine in addition the death-rate for the entire four years of the follow-up period. Some limited comparison can be made in this respect with Shepherd's study (1957), although in his case the follow-up period was five years.

Table 84 shows clearly that the death-rates *per 100 first admissions* in both our units was smaller in these four years of follow-up than the death-rates among Shepherd's patients during the five-year period. It is unlikely that the differences are entirely, or even largely, due to the additional year of follow-up. There are no general population statistics which cover a four-year death-rate, and we cannot relate our figure or those of

TABLE 84

Death-rates during a follow-up period over several years

New Admissions to the Units giving Death-rates per 100 4 Years after Inception		*Admissions to a Mental Hospital giving Death-rates per 100 5 Years after Admission (Shepherd)*	
		1931–3	1945–8
65 years and over	48%	66·7%	64·7%
16–64 years	7%	21·2%	11·6%
All ages	12%	29·7%	26·5%

Shepherd to the general population, but have to express them as a percentage of first admissions.

In the over-sixty-five age-group in our sample the death-rate was 48% for the two units, compared with 66·7% for Shepherd's 1931–3 group and 64·7% for his 1945–8 group. In the younger age-group (sixteen to sixty-four years), the extramural patients again showed up to advantage; we find a death-rate of 7% among the unit patients, compared with 21·2% and 11·6% respectively among Shepherd's two groups. The differences cannot simply be ascribed to the differences in the services as such, but they were at least partly due to the selection that takes place in the intake procedure in these two types of service, as mentioned above.

Table 85 shows, further, that selection of patients at intake is a very important factor, which must not be brushed aside. Here the death-rates are counted separately for a number of periods within the follow-up time. The death-rates are given separately for the first month after inception, the first six months after inception and the first twelve months, and again separately for all the deaths occurring after the first year. The figures in Table 85 show that the rise in mortality in the units and in Shepherd's two groups remain roughly parallel in the first twelve months. After this there is a sharp difference. In Shepherd's groups the mortality drops after the first year, but in the general hospital group the rate continues to rise. Shepherd's figures are in line with Norris's findings (1959, p. 205), which she summarizes thus: '... in the first year, the death-rates

TABLE 85

Proportion of deaths during the follow-up period at various intervals after inception

		Deaths within 1 Month of Admission or Inception	*6 Months*	*12 Months*	*Deaths after 12 Months following Inception or Admission*	*Total Number of Deaths and % of all Admissions*	
Blackpool and Burnley units		11·2%	27·8%	44·5%	55·5%	54	12%
New Admissions to a mental hospital (Shepherd)	1931–3	18·1%	44·8%	59%	40·9%	105	29·7%
	1945–8	38·3%	79·1%	84·3%	15·6%	115	26·5%

for men and women together are over twice as great as those for the second and third years of hospital life', but her rule clearly does not apply to a group of patients in an extramural psychiatric service.

The patients studied by Shepherd and Norris were all in-patient admissions to mental hospital and clearly included a large number of very sick persons, a number of whom could be expected to die within the first hospital year. Those who survived that time approximated more and more to the general population as regards the death-rate. Hence the sharp drop. The extramural psychiatric service, on the other hand, incepted a much more mixed group of patients, including a large number who remained as out-patients from the start, and who were not so seriously ill. In the first year the death-rate could be expected to be only moderately higher than that of the general population and would then continue to rise at something the same rate. There would therefore not be the same steep fall after the first year, as occurred with the mental hospital admissions.

The very important differences amongst the various groups under comparison, however, cannot entirely explain the whole of the marked discrepancy between them, and it seems fairly clear that mortality is at least not any higher for patients who are cared for in an extramural psychiatric service than it is for those admitted to mental hospital.

General Mortality Rate

Death-rates of hospital patients per 1,000 population are only meaningful if they are broken down into age-groups before any comparison with general population figures may be made. This ideal is difficult to reach, as figures for patient-groups are usually too small for this to be effective. Many authors have found themselves thwarted by this predicament (Malzberg, 1934; Shepherd, 1957; Norris, 1959). We met the same difficulty. Nevertheless, we made an attempt to present our figures in an approximately comparable way.

Columns I and II of Table 83 show that the death-rate per 1,000 population during the first year after inception into the units was greater than that in the general population. As the figures in the general population are broken down into age-groups different from those in our sample, we could only compare differences in general trend, but these general trends were quite clear. In every age-group separately the death-rate was several times larger in the patient-group than would be expected in the general population. In the highest age-group (all patients over sixty-five years), the rate was 230·7 per 1,000 population. This is higher even than the rate for those aged eighty-five years and over in the general population, where the figure was 223·2. The sixty to sixty-four age-group of our patients showed a rate nearly nine times that of the general population (135 compared with 15·9). This must surely be very much in excess, particularly as the quoted general population figures do include the fifty-five to sixty age-groups. In the sixteen to fifty-nine age-groups, even the average rate for our patient-group (16·6) was higher than the highest general population rate, where the figures ranged from 0·65 to 15·9 within this age-range.

The general population figures quoted so far refer to the death-rates in England and Wales. We had to choose these figures because those for Lancashire County and for the two catchment areas in particular were not given in the same detail. We only had the crude death-rates here, and indeed these differed from those in England and Wales as a whole. In Lancashire County they were higher: 13·3 per 1,000 population, compared with the figure of 11·6 for England and Wales. Furthermore, the crude death-rates for the respective catchment areas of the two general hospital units were higher still: 17·1 and 17·2.

Thus the difference between the general population rates and those found for our own patients becomes reduced in size, yet when these figures are compared with the crude death-rates of new admissions in our two general hospital units, they are still far below the latter – namely, 51·7 per 1,000 population in the Burnley unit and 46·4 in the Blackpool unit.

In the previous paragraphs we have shown that the death-rate among patients in an extramural general hospital psychiatric service were considerably lower than those amongst mental hospital patients, but it is also clear that patients incepted by any kind of psychiatric service, including the extramural types, have a death-rate far in excess of that in the general

TABLE 86

Crude death-rates

Population	*Crude Death-rate per 1,000 Population (in Cases of Patients within 1 Year of Admission)*
New Admissions to Burnley unit	51·7
General population in the catchment area of Burnley unit	17·1
New Admissions to Blackpool unit	46·4
General population in the catchment area of Blackpool unit	17·2
New Admissions to Blackpool and Burnley units	49
General population of England and Wales	11·6
General population of Lancashire County	13·3
Mental Hospital Admissions in 1931–3 (Shepherd)	161
Mental Hospital Admissions in 1945–8 (Shepherd)	229
Mental Hospital Admissions in 1947–9 (V. Norris)	Men 285 Women 187

population. This is not surprising, since a psychiatric population contains many old and physically ill people, many of them even moribund at the time of admission. Sometimes the illness is concomitant with the mental disorder and very often the mental disorder is a direct expression of the underlying physical illness – for instance, cerebro-vascular disease, toxic state, or cerebral metastases of new growth. Malzberg (1934) is often quoted as saying 'rates of mortality at corresponding ages are three to six times as great among patients with mental disorders as amongst the general population'. It would seem that this estimate comes nearer to our figures than those calculated for the mental hospital populations, which are much in excess of it, i.e. about twenty times as high. Table 86 shows this in relation to the crude death-rates, which in our two units combined are 49 per 1,000 population, nearly three times the rate of the catchment-area general population, where it is 17·2. Rates for the county mental hospital service reported by

Shepherd (1957) were 161 per 1,000 population in the years 1931–3 and 229 in the years 1945–8, while those for the London hospitals quoted by Norris were 187 for females and 265 for males. The latter figures refer to admissions to mental hospital for the years 1947–9. The death-rate for England and Wales at the time of these two studies was approximately 12 per 1,000 population.

Causes of Death

The causes of death based on death certificates are listed in Table 87. They are broken down according to the psychiatric diagnoses at inception to the units. Nearly half of the patients who had died had been admitted in consequence of an organic psychosyndrome; nearly another quarter had had an affective psychosis. The latter is not surprising, as in the sample as a whole the older age-group was rather over-represented amongst the patients with affective psychosis. Our figures are not dissimilar from those of Shepherd (1957), who also found that among those patients who had died the majority had been admitted to hospital showing an organic psychosyndrome. In his study, too, the next largest group among those who died were those patients, like ours, suffering from affective psychosis.

As regards actual causes of death, the most frequent in our group was vascular disease, either cerebral or cardiac (namely, 30%). The two next largest groups were senile dementia and cancer: taken together, they comprised 18% of all deaths. Respiratory diseases, excluding new growth, accounted for 9% and G.P.I. and cerebral tumour for 4% each. Other causes occurring less frequently were renal failure, pancreatitis, etc. The picture is very similar to that found by Shepherd (1957), who found one-third of the deaths of his patients were due to vascular disease, while other conditions severally figured at a 10% rate. In Norris's tables, cerebro-vascular disease heads the list, though her data are not categorized in a strictly comparable way. In her group G.P.I. is prominent as a cause of death, and this is so in Shepherd's group also; it is, however, little represented in our sample, no doubt reflecting the decreased prevalence of this disease over the last twenty to twenty-five years.

TABLE 87

Cause of death as given in death certificate (by diagnosis on inception)

	Organic Psychosyndrome	*Schizophrenia*	*Affective Psychosis*	*Epilepsy*	*Personality Disorder*	*Abnormal Psychogenic Reaction*	*Other*	*Total*
	25	5	11	1	2	6	3	54
Vascular disease	10	2	1	—	1	2	—	16 30%
Senile dementia	7	—	3	—	—	—	—	10 18%
Cancer	4	1	2	—	—	2	1	10 18%
Respiratory disease	1	—	2	—	—	1	1	5 9%
Suicide	—	2	1	—	—	—	—	3 6%
G.P.I.	1	—	—	—	—	—	1	2 4%
Cerebral tumour	1	—	—	1	—	—	—	2 4%
Others or not known	2	—	2	—	1	1	—	6 11%

Suicide

Deaths due to suicide were of particular interest in this context, since a very frequent reason for hospital admission has always been the danger of suicide. Here in an extramural type of service presumably the same patients at risk were not necessarily admitted, and if admitted were soon discharged. Many of them must on the long-term basis be regarded as potential suicidal risks. We found that in fact only 6% of our patients had died in this way.

It is worth noting here that the diagnostic groups most at risk were not the patients suffering from affective psychosis nor from abnormal psychogenic reactions, as one might expect, but the schizophrenics. This becomes more striking if one expresses the figures in terms of rates. Among the schizophrenics the suicide-rate came to 3·2%, while amongst the affective psychoses the figure was 1·4%. One cannot place too much reliance on the significance of this, as the absolute figures are small, but it is well to bear in mind that in an extramural service schizophrenic patients were at least as much, if not more, at risk than patients suffering from a depressive psychosis.

Sainsbury *et al.* (1966) investigated the suicide-rate amongst the patients incepted into an extramural type of service in Chichester. Their concern ran on similar lines to ours and the contention that extramural type of care probably increased the risk of suicide seemed borne out by their findings. They noted that whereas in the first year only 3·7 per 1,000 population had committed suicide, in the second year the figure had risen to 7·4. However, comparison with the conventional mental hospital type of service, based on the Salisbury hospital, showed no such increase. The figures for the latter in the first year were already as high as the Chichester figures in the second year—namely, 7·2 per 1,000 population. Thus the interpretation which suggests itself would be that the extramural type of service in Chichester managed to contain the suicide-rate, but only during the first year; in the second year it reverted to the level found in Salisbury. In our group the overall amount of suicide was rather small. It involved only three patients, which represented only 0·09% of all new inceptions, or one per 1,000 population. In Chichester there were two patients out of 271 who committed suicide, representing 0·74% of all first admissions. The figures are not significantly different and the somewhat higher figure in our group is related to the longer four-year follow-up *versus* the two-year follow-up in Chichester.

If there had been an increased number of suicides among the patients in our own sample, this would surely have shown in the coroners' records for the respective catchment areas and be

TABLE 88

Suicide rates per 1,000 population

Year	*Catchment Area of Burnley Unit*	*Catchment Area of Blackpool Unit*	*England and Wales*	*Chichester Service Area*
1956	0·41	0·18	0·120	*Annual rate*
1957	0·36	0·23	0·122	1952–6
1958	0·32	0·18	0·121	0·13
1959	0·27	0·21	0·118	1959–63
1961	0·23	0·19	0·115	0·14
1962	0·19	0·20	0·121	

reflected in the Census reports in due course. Table 88 compares the official suicide rates in both catchment areas with those for England and Wales as in the Census reports. It can be seen that the suicide-rates in the two catchment areas were considerably higher than for England and Wales; sometimes they appeared twice as high. Sainsbury *et al.* (1966) have calculated the suicide-rates per 1,000 population on the coroners' records for those who had been patients at the hospital. Sainsbury also reports the rate for Chichester, but in this case it is an annual rate. It amounts to 0·137 per 1,000 for the years 1959–63, which is slightly higher than the figures shown in our table for England and Wales, but lower than for the catchment areas of our two general hospital units, and particularly so when compared with the Burnley unit. It will be remembered that the suicide-rate for Burnley was shown in the Census to top the list for all the areas in England and Wales. The object in making these assessments, for Sainsbury as for ourselves, was to see whether the suicide-rate would be affected by the introduction of the new psychiatric service in the area. For both places, Chichester and our two northern areas, Burnley and Blackpool, the findings were reassuring. In Chichester the annual rate for the years 1952–6, before the new service was introduced, was insignificantly smaller (0·13 per 1,000) than in the subsequent period. In our own case, there was no significant rise between the figures previous to 1959, and those after; if anything, the Burnley figures show a steady decline, while in Blackpool the figures pursue a fluctuating course. The findings are reassuring. It is true this is an indirect way of assessing the effect of an extramural service on the suicide-rate and may be misleading, since such relatively small numbers are involved. Yet the figures as they stand do not suggest an increased suicide-rate, and indeed, if the extramural service affects the rate at all, it has to be seen in the direction of a slight decrease.

Clinical and Social Aspects of Mortality

In what way did this group of patients who died after inception differ from the survivors, and what were their special characteristics, if any? To answer these questions we selected a random sample from the rest of the patients, which we then used as a control group for the group who had died.

In most respects the patients who died were similar to the controls, the notable exception being the patient's age. The fact that there was no difference in sex distribution in the two groups contrasts with the findings of both Norris and Shepherd in regard to the mental hospital admissions, both of these investigators finding an excess of male mortality. 70% of those who died in the sample were over sixty years of age, whereas in the controls the older age-group constituted only 22%. This was an expected finding. Men and women appeared, however, in the same proportion in both age-groups, both among the dead and among the controls. Other factors, such as whether the patient lived alone or with the family, did not seem related to the death-rate in any way. The majority of those who died had been living as members of a family group, and very few were long-stay members of any institution or hostel or hotel; and the same situation was found among the controls. The marital status of the patients did not show any relationship to death-rates either, nor did social class, with the exception of Social Class II, which seemed to be over-represented among the dead ($p < 0{\cdot}02$). Thus social deprivation, as would be engendered by lonely living or poverty, did not seem to have affected our sample and, if anything, the more affluent social group seemed more at risk.

The relationship to diagnosis has already been discussed and was shown in Table 87. Patients who were suffering from an organic psychosyndrome at inception, as one might expect, comprised 50% of the group who died as compared with 4% of the controls. As vascular disease was the most common cause of death, it must be assumed that the organic psychosyndromes were in many cases due to cerebral vascular disease, and that in these cases the cause of the psychosyndrome was also the cause of death. Schizophrenia was conspicuous because of its low death rate (9·3%) and, allowing for the two suicides, it becomes even lower. Among the controls the proportion of schizophrenics was 24%. Personality disorders also showed a low death-rate. They were represented by only 3·8% among the dead and by 34% among the controls. The affective psychoses were represented equally among the dead and the controls (20%).

With the exception of the organic psychosyndromes, the difference in diagnostic distribution was probably due to the age-distribution. Schizophrenia and personality disorder arose predominantly in the younger age-groups, whereas a larger percentage of older patients appeared among the affective psychoses. Many of the abnormal psychogenic reactions had an exacerbated non-psychiatric disease accompanying them, independently of the psychiatric disorder which had brought about inception.

A large number of the patients who died did in fact have non-psychiatric disease also present at inception. By this we mean physical illness other than that underlying the organic psychosyndrome. The percentage of those who suffered from such additional disorder at inception was 42·6%, very much in excess of what we found in the controls, where the figure was 14% for those who had such illness ($p < 0{\cdot}001$). If one adds physical illness which arose after inception, the differences become yet greater. Thus the patients who died were undoubtedly a very sick group at inception with a high morbidity rate throughout the four years.

The Burden on the Services

(*a*) *Medical Services*

Although a large proportion of the patients who died did so early within the follow-up period, the majority lived on for a considerable time right on to the fourth year. These patients, often suffering from severe terminal illness, might be expected to place an extra burden on the various medical services. Comparison with our controls, however, showed that the usage between the two groups was similar. The slight differences found were as follows: among the group that died, more were initially incepted by domiciliary visits than among the controls, who tended to come more as out-patients. As many as 50% of the patients who died had been incepted by domiciliary visits compared with 24% of the controls, but only 31·5% of them came as out-patients, compared with 56% of the controls ($p < 0{\cdot}01$). This reflects the high incidence of non-psychiatric illness in this group and the tendency for its members to belong to the higher age-group. The same factors were probably responsible for the result that more of the patients who died were initially admitted as in-patients than was the case among the controls. Here, however, the difference between the group that died (69%) and the controls (60%) was barely significant.

The usage of the psychiatric services during the four-year period was very similar in the two groups, except that those who died had more in-patient admissions to the units and to the mental hospital. In-patient admission was more frequently resorted to probably because once again of the serious nature of the physical condition of the patients rather than the abnormality of their mental state as such. Thus, of the patients who subsequently died, 81·5% were admitted to the units, compared with 62% of the controls ($p < 0{\cdot}02$). Although there were more frequent admissions, it did not lead to prolonged stay. The total in-patient time is exactly the same in the two groups, which means that while there were more frequent admissions, there were more frequent discharges and the length of stay on each occasion was correspondingly brief. Those who later died tended to stay for shorter periods; for instance, 44% stayed for less that one month in all, as compared with 30% of the controls. Admission to the mental hospitals on the other hand were equally frequent in the two groups and amounted to about 20%. Those who subsequently died tended to stay longer than was the case with the controls (12% of them stayed up to one year, compared with 4% of the controls).

One can say that the psychiatric services were used by the two groups in a slightly different way, but, quantitatively speaking, not to excess in either case. What was more surprising was that the group who died, with so many organic psycho-syndromes and with so much non-psychiatric illness among them, did not use the general hospitals more than the controls, whether as in-patients or out-patients. (In fact, less than 10% so attended.) As regards the in-patient stay in general hospital, this tended to show the same pattern as with the psychiatric beds in the units, i.e. more frequent admission of the group that died (40%) as compared with the controls (22%), while the aggregate length of stay remained the same for both groups.

Lastly, it is interesting to find that not even the general practitioner had markedly more dealings with the group that died than with the control group: 44% of the former had frequent or regular contacts with their doctor as compared with 38% of the controls. ('Frequent' here means 'two to six consultations in six months', while 'regular' means 'at least once a month'.)

(*b*) *Social Services*

We compared the two groups as to whether they had received an equal amount of social agency care throughout the four years. We found that this was so to practically the same extent: 35% of those who died received such care, compared with 31% of the controls. They also received constant care slightly more often, but the differences did not reach statistical significance.

The Burden on the Household

Following the procedure described above (p. 97), we proceeded to assess the 'objective' burden carried by the households in the two groups. There seemed no difference between the patients who died and the controls as regards financial loss to the household and the amount of nursing care required, which is perhaps a little surprising when we consider the amount of illness present in those who died. There was naturally less separation from young children in this group than in the control group, no doubt due in part to the higher proportion of older people among those who died.

When we turn to the 'subjective' burden, however, there were some very marked differences between the two groups. Severe 'subjective' burden was complained of in 27% of the households of those who had died, but among the controls, the proportion was only 9%. The figures for 'some' burden were 55% and 38% respectively. Finally, where the patients had died, there were only 18% of the families who had sensed no burden, whereas for the controls the figure was as high as 53%. The differences are highly significant ($p < 0{\cdot}001$).

We have seen, therefore, that the 'objective' burden on the household was very similar in the two groups, but 'subjective' complaints of a severe kind were made much more frequently by the relatives of those who died. Perhaps this reflects the distress caused by being closely related to a severely physically ill person during the terminal illness. Perhaps also the extramural service was in some way less helpful to this particular group of patients than it might have been, in so far as 'subjective' burden was experienced to a so much greater degree by the families with moribund patients than by the controls. It seems that no greater amount of social agency care was invoked either and, as we shall see in the next section, there was a higher incidence of personal complaint about the units and the management of the case than occurred with the controls. Can it be that the psychiatric extramural services do not make the moribund patient sufficiently their concern?

Attitudes

It must first be noted that, despite the high degree of 'subjective' burden in the households of those who died, the *majority* had no complaints to make about the units (76% as compared with 83% among the controls). Minor complaints amounted to 12% and 14% respectively; yet there were a minority of informants who remained definitely dissatisfied. Either they had serious complaints to make against the units (12% as compared with 3% of the controls, $p < 0{\cdot}01$), or they considered that treatment had been inappropriate (20%, compared with 10% of the controls), or they felt that something more should have been done (7%, compared with 8% of the controls). The latter differences are not significant.

We also asked relatives what difference in-patient admissions had made to the household. In 64% of the households of those who had died and in 56% of the controls, the relatives expressed gratitude for admission and said there had been great relief to the household. The remainder (in almost equal proportions in the two groups) seemed indifferent, but in no case had admission created any particular difficulty. It seemed, therefore, that hospital admission brings great relief equally whether patients are suffering from their terminal physical illness or whether they are mentally ill without any particular physical complication. There appeared to be no objection to the patients not being nursed at home during this terminal illness. When the question of admission to mental hospital was raised, the proportion of those in favour and those against was the same in both groups, a ratio of four in favour to one against, indicating that the prejudice against mental hospital admission was but little more than that against hospital admission generally, even for patients with terminal illness (Hoenig *et al.*, 1966).

Conclusions

Although this group of patients who died during the four-year follow-up were on the whole not a heavy burden on the psychiatric, general medical, or social services, as compared with other psychiatric patients, their families do seem to have borne a considerable brunt, and complained rather more of this than the families in our control group. They would appear, therefore, to be a sub-group of patients well worth further scrutiny to see how the extramural service might extend them and their families better help.

(IV) USAGE OF MENTAL HOSPITAL

So far we have looked at the services provided by the two general hospital psychiatric units and tried to estimate the success of their work in terms of their declared policy, particularly as regards their success in avoiding admission of patients to mental hospital. Our findings have shown that they did indeed succeed to an impressive degree in achieving this goal – to an impressive degree, but not completely. Out of the total sample of 273 new patients 6·2% were admitted to mental hospitals on inception and another 13·4% were so admitted in the course of the subsequent four years.

Allowing for the position of the Blackpool unit with its more restricted number of beds, these figures may appear small enough as 'failures' in terms of the stated policy. However, 'failures of policy' are always worth studying, and more perhaps may be learnt from them than from the 'successes' themselves. In this section we shall endeavour to look into the factors which played a role in diverting this small group of patients into mental hospital care, despite avowed efforts to the contrary.

Number of Patients Admitted

The number of patients sent to mental hospital differed in the two units. Table 89 shows the admission figures in each case. It will be remembered that the two units differed in size. The Burnley unit had 0·4 beds per 1,000 population and during the four years admitted 5·8% of its patients to mental hospital. This figure can be broken down further in that in the course of the four years 5% were admitted to the unit itself as well as to the mental hospital, whereas only 0·8% were admitted to mental hospital alone. Most of the patients that made up the 5% had been admitted to the unit first and only entered mental hospital subsequently. In the Blackpool unit, on the other hand, which had only about one-third of the number of beds at its disposal (0·15 beds per 1,000 population), 30% of the patients were at some time admitted to mental hospital. The difference between this and the Burnley figure is highly significant ($p < 0{\cdot}001$). Moreover, the proportion of patients who went to the mental

TABLE 89

Type of in-patient admission
(by units)

	In-patients			*No In-patient Treatment (including not known or not applicable)*	*Total*	
	Mental Hospital Only	*Mental Hospital and Unit*	*Unit Only*			
Blackpool unit, 0·15 beds per 1,000 population	10·4%	19·6%	40%	30%	153	100%
Burnley unit, 0·47 beds per 1,000 population	0·8%	5%	69·2%	25%	120	100%
Both units	6·2%	13·4%	52·6%	27·8%	273	100%

hospital without any unit in-patient treatment was much higher too – namely, 10·4% – while 19·6% were in-patients at the unit and at the mental hospital as well.

The question that suggests itself is whether these differences between the two units were due to more in-patient admissions in general in the Blackpool area, but this can be quickly dismissed. If one looks at the respective samples as a whole, there appears to be no significant difference anywhere between them in the percentage who were never admitted as in-patients, neither to unit nor mental hospital. It will be remembered that in the Blackpool area 30% and in the Burnley area 25% never had any in-patient treatment at all – or, if looked at the other way round, 70–75% of the patients in both units had in-patient treatment at some time. If one takes initial disposal only into account, the figures are even closer: 58% in Blackpool and 61% in-patients in Burnley.

It would seem that when in-patient treatment was required, the Burnley unit could make more use of its own beds, whereas the Blackpool unit was forced to divert a larger proportion of patients to the mental hospital. During the subsequent four years, the Burnley unit admitted 69·2% of the patients to its own beds and the Blackpool unit only 40% ($p < 0{\cdot}01$). The reason for this different usage of unit and mental hospital beds was obviously the above-mentioned shortage of beds at the Blackpool unit, and the relatively larger deflection of in-patients to the mental hospital must be understood as an overflow phenomenon. The psychiatrist at the Blackpool unit simply had to resort to mental hospital admission more frequently because he had no vacant beds in the unit to accommodate the demand for in-patient admission. The slight difference in the overall percentage of in-patient admissions (namely, 70% in Blackpool and 75% in Burnley) can also be seen perhaps as further evidence for the fact that the Blackpool unit had far less room in which to manœuvre. It would seem that, where flexibility of choice was still possible, the Blackpool unit preferred to try to manage their patients as out-patients rather than send them to mental hospital, though the indications for this were only of the small order of 5%.

Further evidence that the higher mental hospital admissions in the Blackpool area were merely due to shortage of unit beds comes from the fact that the stay in mental hospital was only for a very short duration. Table 90 shows that whereas the medium-stay groups (i.e. from four to twelve months) were of approximately equal size (2·6% in the Blackpool area, 1·1% in the Burnley area), the short-stay groups (under three months'

TABLE 90

Aggregate length of in-patient treatment in mental hospital

	None	*Up to 3 Months*	*4–12 Months*	*Over 1 Year*	*Total*
Blackpool unit	68%	21·8%	2·6%	7·6%	100%
Burnley unit	92%	5·8%	1·1%	1·1%	100%
Total	79·5%	14%	2%	4·5%	100%

stay) were much more numerous in the Blackpool area – in fact, almost four times as numerous (21·8% in the Blackpool area and 5·2% in the Burnley area). This seems to show that while the Blackpool psychiatrist had to send more patients to mental hospital, he tended to make use of these beds for short-stay purposes only, very much as the beds were being used in the general hospital psychiatric units. One might conclude that had both units been of equal size, the figures would have turned out very much the same.

Comment seems called for as regards the differences between the two units in respect of the longer-term patients (over one-year stay). Table 90 shows that whereas in the Blackpool area the figure was 7·6%, in the Burnley area only 1·1% were longer-stay mental hospital patients. Earlier on (p. 67) we speculated that mental hospital stay as such might cause more prolonged hospital stay, at least in some cases. Certainly the possibility cannot be dismissed. But our analysis of the difference in the two units, which is clearly linked with discharge rates, suggests that this would not have been the only factor; it seems that certain social differences in the two catchment areas need to be taken into account also. In the Burnley area there was a more settled population and the families were able to give the patient better support. Discharge from mental hospital could be arranged more easily. The population of the Blackpool area showed a greater mobility and the niche to which the patient might return from hospital tended to disappear. Thus the patients in the Blackpool area tended to spend more time in hospital, though other factors no doubt were operating as well. It has to be borne in mind that the above percentages refer to the 'total hospital time', i.e. they represent an aggregate stay over the four years. Some patients therefore who appear in the longer-stay group only fall into this group because of an accumulation of repeated short stays.

The general administrative conclusion that could be drawn from these observations would seem to be that the policy of avoiding mental hospital admission can only be achieved if the psychiatric units in the general hospitals have a certain minimum number of beds at their disposal; 0·4 beds per 1,000 population, which was the number available in the Burnley area, appears to be such a minimum. It is true that even in Burnley a number of admissions to the mental hospital took place over the four years, but, as pointed out in Chapter III, the unit beds were not being used exclusively by patients from the catchment area at this time: in fact, they served a good number of patients from outside this area, although these latter were formally excluded from our investigation.

It is also reasonable to expect that there will always remain a certain number of patients difficult to accommodate in a general hospital setting, and their needs will have to be catered for in some other institution, mental hospital, or unit dealing with special cases, e.g. patients who are maximum security risks, certain types of addicts, etc. It is remarkable that the overall bed usage is so constant in the two units, even though in the Blackpool area the psychiatrist had to deal with the added difficulty of finding mental hospital beds for the overflow.

Factors influencing Admission

Irrespective of bed resources, some selection had to operate which led to mental hospital admission for the patients rather than admission to the units, and it seems justifiable to examine the two units jointly to elicit what factors were involved in bringing such a selection about.

TABLE 91

Type of in-patient admission by sex

	In-patients			*No In-patient Treatment*	*Total*
	Mental Hospital Only	*Mental Hospital and Unit*	*Unit Only*		
Male	9 7·6%	21 17·8%	52 44%	36 30·6%	118 100%
Female	8 5·2%	15 9·7%	92 59·2%	40 25·9%	155 100%
Tota	17	36	144	76	273

TABLE 92

Type of in-patient admission by age-groups

	In-patients			*No In-patient Treatment*	*Total*
	Mental Hospital Only	*Mental Hospital and Unit*	*Unit Only*		
Under 60 years	15 8·2%	28 15·2%	80 43·5%	61 33·1%	184 100%
Over 60 years	2 2·2%	8 9%	64 72%	15 16·8%	89 100%

For this purpose we divided the total sample into four groups: (1) those who were admitted to mental hospital only, (2) those admitted at one time or other to the unit and the mental hospital, (3) those admitted to the unit only, and (4) those who had never been in-patients at all. We then compared the four groups in relation to a number of factors.

Sex and Age

Of the male patients 25·4% went into mental hospital (including those who went both to unit and mental hospital), whereas of the women patients only 14·9% were so admitted ($p < 0{\cdot}05$). The figures also show that although men and women were equally admitted to the units (taking all unit admissions, exclusive or not) a large proportion of men were subsequently admitted to the mental hospital (17·8%); the figure for the women was only 9·5% ($p < 0{\cdot}05$). This suggests that although an equal attempt had been made to keep patients of both sexes in the unit in preference to the mental hospital, nevertheless it seems to have proved more difficult to keep male patients in the unit when readmission became necessary.

The situation regarding *age* of the patients was slightly more complex. The older patients (over sixty years) showed a higher admission rate in general than the younger group (irrespective of whether admission was to unit or mental hospital). 83·2% of the over-sixty group became in-patients at some time during the four years, whereas only 66·9% of the under-sixty group did so. However, 72% of the older patients continued to have unit treatment exclusively and only 9% subsequently went to the mental hospital, whereas in the under-sixty age-group only 43·5% remained unit in-patients exclusively and 15·2% found their way subsequently to mental hospital. Even among those patients who received all their in-patient treatment in the mental hospital, the same trend is apparent. Of the over-sixty age-group only 2·2% fell into this group, while the figure for the under-sixty group was 8·2%.

These figures show that the general hospital psychiatric units were better able to accommodate the older age-group, despite the fact that such patients made a higher demand on beds than the younger group. This finding is particularly encouraging,

TABLE 93

Type of admission
(by diagnosis)

	In-patient						*No In-patient Treatment*		*Total*	
	Mental Hospital Only		*Mental Hospital and Unit*		*Unit Only*					
Organic psychosyndrome	3	8·1%	5	13·5%	24	67·6%	4	10·8%	36	100%
Schizophrenia	8	12·9%	19	30·6%	22	35·5%	13	21%	62	100%
Affective psychosis	1	1·5%	3	4·4%	48	70·5%	16	23·6%	68	100%
Personality disorder	4	5·8%	7	10·1%	31	45%	27	39·1%	69	100%
Abnormal psychogenic reaction		—	2	9%	10	45·5%	10	45·5%	22	100%
Others	1	6%		—	9	56%	6	38%	16	100%

because most of the misgivings in the minds of critics of predominantly extramural psychiatric care are concerned with this geriatric group of patients. It is felt that, because they tend to suffer from chronic illnesses and from the social problems that surround ageing, they might not be adequately contained within such a service. The fact is that in this respect they seemed to be rather less of a problem than the younger age-groups of psychiatric patients.

Clinical Factors

Of the various clinical factors that might have influenced the situation, diagnosis obviously needed to be considered. Its effect on hospital admission is illustrated in Table 93. The relationships are somewhat complex. The lowest demand for in-patient beds in general came from the patients with abnormal psychogenic reactions (54·5%) or personality disorders (60·9%). The figures for patients with affective psychoses were 76·4% and for those with schizophrenia 79%. The highest rate of all (89·2%) fell to the patients suffering from an organic psychosyndrome. Most of the admissions were to the units, and altogether very few went to the mental hospital exclusively. Substantial percentages were found only amongst the schizophrenics (12·9%) and the organic psychosyndromes (8·1%).

As regards all mental hospital admissions during the four years, the schizophrenics formed certainly far and away the largest group (43·5%). The figures for the other diagnostic groupings ranged from 5·9% up to 21·9%. The difference is significant ($p < 0{\cdot}01$).

A smaller percentage of the schizophrenics (35·5%), on the other hand, were treated as unit in-patients only, contrasting, for instance, with the groups suffering from organic psychosyndromes (67·6%) and from affective psychoses (70·5%) ($p < 0{\cdot}01$). It appears that not only did the schizophrenic patients require a high degree of hospitalization in general, second only to the patients with organic psychosyndromes, but they tended to be admitted to mental hospital more than the other diagnostic groups, both initially and after treatment in the units.

Another relevant factor might be thought to be the length of

TABLE 94

Type of in-patient admission (by duration of illness before inception)

Duration of Illness before Inception	In-patients				No In-patient Treatment		Total	
	Mental Hospital		Unit only					
Up to 2 years	20	13%	96	62%	39	25%	155	100%
2 years and over	33	28%	48	40%	37	32%	118	100%

the patient's illness both before inception and through the follow-up period. This was indeed so as regards illness before inception, particularly where it had lasted more than two years. 28% of these chronic patients were sent into mental hospital as compared with only 13% of those who had been ill for shorter time ($p < 0{\cdot}001$). The less-chronic patients were mostly treated in the unit (62% of them in the unit as compared with 40% of the chronic group ($p < 0{\cdot}001$). This is not unexpected. It suggests that patients ill long before inception at the unit, who had perhaps had treatment elsewhere, including in-patient treatment, were felt now to be less responsive to active treatment methods and accordingly were not admitted as in-patients to the units at all. This was so for 32% of the more chronic patients as compared with 25% of the less chronic group. If admission was thought necessary, this tended to be in slightly greater numbers to the mental hospital. While this was the

TABLE 95

Types of in-patient admission (by morbidity during 4 years)

Duration of Morbidity during the follow-up Period	In-patients				No In-patient Treatment		Total	
	Mental Hospital		Unit Only					
Under 1 year	9	14·6%	36	58%	17	27·4%	62	100%
Over 1 year	41	35%	58	57%	16	14%	115	100%

trend, it must not be overlooked that, nevertheless, the units took on a sizeable proportion of the patients in any case – namely, 40%. While, then, the duration of the patient's illness before inception exerted considerable influence, the extent to which the patient remained ill after inception was less of a factor. There seemed a slight but significant tendency for admission to mental hospital to occur more often with those patients who showed an aggregate duration of illness of more than one year (i.e. for more than 25% of the follow-up period). The figures here were 35% for the more chronically ill, compared with 14·6% for the more quickly recoverable patients ($p < 0{\cdot}01$)

TABLE 96

Type of in-patient admission
(by clinical features: danger to others)

Has been a danger to others	*In-patients*			*No In-patient Treatment*	*Total*
	Mental Hospital Only	*Mental Hospital and Unit*	*Unit Only*		
Never or only occasionally	4·4%	9·6%	59·6%	26·5%	100%
Periodically or constantly	14·7%	41·2%	38·2%	5·9%	100%

Following the method described in an earlier chapter (p. 97), we examined the disturbing behaviour shown by the patients during the four years of follow-up. The only behaviour that seemed to show any particular correlation with mental hospital admission was 'behaviour dangerous to the self and/or others'. Only 5·9% of the patients showing this constantly or periodically were treated as out-patients during the four-year period, compared with 26·5% of those who never showed this behaviour or did so only occasionally. Only 14% of this latter group went to mental hospital; the great majority (59·6%) received treatment as in-patients in the units exclusively. But of the former group who showed this type of disturbing behaviour more markedly through the four years, 55·9% went at some time to mental hospital and only 38·2% stayed as unit in-patients exclusively. It would seem that this type of patient was rather more difficult to manage on an out-patient basis alone, nor did the general hospital psychiatric unit tolerate them so readily as in-patients. The relative figures are shown in Table 96.

TABLE 97

Type of in-patient admission
(by clinical features: hypochondriasis)

Has shown Hypochondriasis	*In-patients*			*No In-patient Treatment*	*Total*
	Mental Hospital Only	*Mental Hospital and Unit*	*Unit Only*		
No	7·5%	13%	55·2%	24·3%	100%
Yes, but mild only	—	12·5%	69%	18·5%	100%
Yes, severe	—	8·5%	83%	8·5%	100%

Grad *et al.* (1963) found admission rates affected by the amount of hypochondriasis displayed by patients. With our patients this symptom occurred in only 9·8% of the cases, and it was therefore not easy to assess its influence, if any. It certainly seemed to exercise some pressure towards hospitalization as such. Only 18·5% of patients with this symptom to a mild degree remained out-patients as compared with 24·3% of the patients without it, but the difference is not statistically significant. When hospitalization did arise, however, it tended to be to the units rather than to the mental hospital, and certainly none of our hypochondriacal patients was admitted to mental hospital exclusively; only two patients (12·5%) went to mental hospital after being treated in the unit, while 69% of them were unit in-patients only. If we take only the most severe cases into account, the trend becomes clearer. Of the twelve patients who showed this symptom severely and constantly 83% were in-patients at the units, 8·5% had mental hospital treatment as well, and 8·5% remained as out-patients. Thus while hypochondriasis seemed associated with hospitalization to a considerable degree, the symptom did not appear to lead to mental hospital admission rather than to the units. The complex figures are shown in Table 97, above.

TABLE 98

Type of in-patient admission (by social class)

Social Class	*In-patients*		*No In-patient Treatment*	*Total*
	Mental Hospital	*Unit Only*		
I and II	23%	54%	23%	100%
III	18%	54%	28%	100%
IV	13%	51%	36%	100%
V	35%	39%	26%	100%

Social Factors

Social class had no marked effect on hospital admission. The general rates in this respect (with unit and mental hospital admission taken together) did not show much difference, the percentage varying from 64% to 78%. The admission rates to mental hospital ranged from 13% to 23%, with the exception of Social Class V, where the figure was 35%. The difference, however, proved to be only just significant ($p < 0{\cdot}05$). Thus the actual social class to which the patients belonged appeared to influence the position very little, whether there was mental hospital admission or not: a reassuring finding, perhaps, after the emphasis that is sometimes laid on the social discrimination found in relation to mental hospital admission and on the varying treatments accorded patients, e.g. by Hollinshead and Redlich (1962) and others.

The patient's civil status, on the other hand, did seem to exert some influence, as shown below in Table 99. We can see that slightly more single patients became in-patients in general (75% as compared with 69·5% of the married patients). But single patients showed a much higher admission rate to mental hospital (34% as compared with 12·5% of the married patients, $p < 0{\cdot}001$). Patients with family ties did not have to be

TABLE 99

Type of in-patient admission
(by marital status)

Marital State	*In-patients*			*No In-patient Treatment*	*Total*
	Mental Hospital Only	*Mental Hospital and Unit*	*Unit Only*		
Married	4·4%	8·1%	57%	30·5%	100%
Single	10·5%	23·5%	41%	25%	100%
Widowed, separated, divorced	5·4%	13·5%	59·5%	21·6%	100%

admitted so frequently, and when so admitted they tended to stay as unit in-patients rather than enter mental hospital, while the reverse was true for single patients. The widowed, separated, or divorced tended to form an intermediary group. They paralleled the single patients when in-patient admissions in general were concerned (78·4%), but in the case of mental hospital admissions they were far fewer, the figure being only 18·9%. No doubt more family support was forthcoming than for the single patient, but not as much as for the married patients.

It seems possible that the family group exercised a protective effect but it is not easy to demonstrate this clearly. For instance, if hospital admissions are scrutinized according to the size of the patients' households, the relationship does not seem a simple one at all. Once the household goes beyond five members, there is a slight difference in hospital admission, but the differences do not reach statistical significance. Simply to assess the size of the household is too crude a method to get at the emotional ties which might have protective influence or, as Brown *et al* (1962) have argued, might have the opposite effect: 'the more emotionally involved the patient was with those with whom he shared the household, the more readily was he returned to hospital'. The 'face-to-face confrontation' often had a crisis-producing effect. In Brown's study, of course, the investigation was concerned with schizophrenic patients only. It is fair to add that his findings have not been borne out by other investigators (e.g.

Kelly, 1964; Waters and Northorer, 1965). In our own sample only 9·1% of the patients from households of more than five members had mental hospital admission as compared with 15.6% to 22·3% in the case of smaller households. But the differences are not statistically significant.

TABLE 100

Type of in-patient admission
(by 'subjective' burden)

'Subjective' Burden	*In-patients*		*No In-patient Treatment*	*Total*
	Mental Hospital	*Unit Only*		
None	8·6%	60%	31·4%	100%
Some	25%	57%	18%	100%
Severe ...	28%	60%	12%	100%

'Subjective' Burden on the Household

The burden felt by the patient's family or household has some influence on mental hospital admissions, as Grad *et al.* (1963) have shown elsewhere. The same trend in our own sample can be seen in Table 100. Of those patients whose families reported no 'subjective' burden at all over the four years, only 8·6% were ever admitted to mental hospital, whereas 25% of those patients whose families complained of some burden and 28% of those where burden was felt to be severe did find their way into mental hospital. These differences are significant ($p < 0 \cdot 01$). Mental hospital admission can be regarded as one way of relieving the pressure felt by households who carry a sick person in their midst. In our sample when pressure became severe mental hospital admission was resorted to in many cases as the first step. This is shown by the figures relating to those who went to mental hospital exclusively, without having a general hospital bed. The patients whose families complained of severe burden were found in this group five times as often (20%) compared with 3·7% and 14·2% respectively where the families either complained not at all or complained only of moderate burden.

This gradient is in the expected direction and the differences are again significant (p <0·01).

Not only the decision as to whether the patient should go to mental hospital rather than to the unit, but also whether he should be retained as an out-patient seemed influenced by this factor of 'subjective' burden felt by the household. Table 100 shows that the more severe the 'subjective' burden, the less likely it was that the patient would remain an out-patient; where there was no burden at all, the figure for out-patient treatment is as high as 31·4%; it drops to 18% where some burden had been complained of, and where severe burden had been endured it drops yet further to 12%.

It seems noteworthy, however, that the 'subjective' burden felt by the households did not correlate at all with in-patient admission to the general hospital psychiatric units, the figure being *c.* 60% for all categories (no, some, and severe burden). In-patient admission to the unit seems therefore to have been a straightforward therapeutic measure – that is, determined by medical considerations only – and was not determined significantly by any particular burden created for the household. It was apparently more a clinical decision than one based on the assessment of the social circumstances to which the patient's illness had given rise.

TABLE 101

Type of in-patient admission
(by social agency care given)

Social Agency Care given	*In-patients*		*No In-patient Treatment*	*Total*
	Mental Hospital	*Unit Only*		
No	10·9%	56·5%	32·6%	100%
Yes	30·9%	54·1%	15%	100%

Social Agency Care

The distress felt by the patient's household was also reflected in the demands made by the families on the social agencies. The patients who received social agency care were admitted to mental hospital more frequently – namely, in 30% of the cases, compared with 10·9% in those who had no social agency care. Only 15% of those who had received help remained out-patients, whereas in the other group it was 32·6% ($p < 0{\cdot}01$). Exclusive admission to the units occurred with equal frequency, irrespective of whether social agency care had been received or not (see Table 101). As we have pointed out earlier, mental hospital admissions were usually multiple through the four years, with patients often staying only short periods and moving in and out a good deal, so that the figures of social agency care probably reflect the continuing need of the families during the periods when the patients were out of hospital. Taken in conjunction with all the foregoing, the figures suggest that social agency care did seem to have been directed to those who needed it most. Surely this is quite gratifying?

Those patients who went to mental hospital, but whose household did not receive any social care, were further analysed. There seemed presumptive evidence that they came from households where such care might be needed, and it seemed important to investigate why they had failed to receive any. The group was a small one in absolute figures (fourteen patients in all) and we attempted to find out why no social care had been given in every case. We found that in four-fifths there had in fact been no need for any social agency care, or so the households had felt, rightly or wrongly. We are reporting the views of the relatives concerned and these might not have been the view of the outside observer. Nevertheless, these households claimed that they had not felt the lack of social agency care during the four years, which was a different view from that of the remaining fifth, who felt they had been in need, but had been reluctant to ask, or else did not know how to obtain help. This small group of people, needing help but somehow failing to get it, is of particular interest to those who organize this aspect of the mental health services, because there is perhaps some room for improvement. That they present a real problem is suggested by the fact that they are found particularly in this group of fourteen persons who came to be admitted to mental hospital and had constituted a problem which the units were unable to handle; but we also find them in the same proportion (*c.* 10%)

in the households of patients treated as unit in-patients, and even amongst those patients who remained as out-patients throughout, showing that the problem is more widespread than with the mental hospital patients alone.

Attitudes of Patients and Relatives

Operational research into services, as we have previously suggested, is incomplete unless some insight is gained into the attitudes of those who in fact use these services. At the time of inception at the unit the following opinions prevailed: 47% of our patients had no objection to being admitted to the psychiatric unit, yet as many as 53% expressed some misgivings over the step. Perhaps it was not surprising that there still seemed such a high incidence of reluctance to enter a psychiatric unit, even though it was located in the nearby general hospital. Unfortunately, in spite of much progress, the public continue to attach some stigma to psychiatric admission wherever it may be. But it was rather surprising to find that the reluctance found amongst the patients to be admitted to mental hospital was no higher – in fact, somewhat lower – than that felt about admission to the new type of in-patient service. 44% of the patients were reluctant for mental hospital admission, as can be seen from Table 102.

TABLE 102

Attitudes to in-patient admission to unit or mental hospital

Attitude at Inception	*Patient*		*Relatives*
	To Unit	*To Mental Hospital*	*To Mental Hospital*
Content	47%	56·2%	78%
Reluctant	53%	43·8%	22%

The relatives on the other hand tended to show even less prejudice than the patients against mental hospital admission. 78% of them were in favour of such admission and only 22% declared themselves against it. Since the attitude of the relatives towards mental hospital admission was coloured by their particular relationship to the patient, the permissive attitude to mental hospital admission might well reflect the pressure under which the households lived when the patient was at home. The difficulties had been such that mental hospital admissions seemed a reasonable way out, and it had been the habitual way out before the units had been established. The figures reflect in fact the 'subjective' burden. This seemed indeed to play some part in whether patients were admitted to mental hospital or not in the course of the four years. Where 'subjective' burden was present but no objection to mental hospital admission existed on the part of the household, 79% of the patients were admitted to mental hospital and 12·6% to the unit, but when objections were voiced (in one-fifth of the cases – 22%), not a single case was admitted to mental hospital.

The attitudes of the relatives, however, seemed to have changed in the course of the four years. At the end of the follow-up time more of them had reservations about mental hospital admission. In fact 44% expressed themselves against it as compared with 22% at the beginning. This rise in the proportion of those who objected was observed not only among those families where the patient has been in mental hospital through the four years, but occurred even when the patient had been treated in the unit exclusively. Thus one can see a swing of public opinion away from the original permissive attitude to mental hospital admission towards a preference for general hospital admission, as people become more familiar with the work of the units. When fresh opportunities exist, more and more of the public expect treatment to take place in the new establishments. This is not so much an increase of prejudice against the older mental hospital, but an appreciation of new and convenient alternatives, which had not been available before.

Asked at the end of the four years whether they had considered the management of the patient's illness appropriate, 87·6% of the informants thought this had been so, and only 12·6% had certain reservations on the point. This attitude seemed to depend to an extent on where the patient had in fact been admitted. Where there had been mental hospital admission, 21% of the relatives expressed themselves as dissatisfied, but when there had been treatment in the unit exclusively, only 8% expressed themselves thus. It did not seem to mean, however, that the informants were resenting admission to psychiatric beds as such, as a similar amount of dissatisfaction was expressed when the patients had remained as out-patients only (20%). Finally, both patients and their relatives were asked if in their opinion more could have been done to help them. 5·5% of the patients and 9·5% of the informants did indeed think so, but admission to mental hospital seemed in no way to affect the opinion. The vast majority of the patients (94·5%) and of the relatives (90·5%) felt that the help they had derived from the service had been all that could have been given.

Conclusions

We have now reviewed the main factors which correlated with mental hospital admission and appeared to determine to some extent whether a patient would fall into the minority who, even in a predominantly extramural service, nevertheless find themselves admitted to a mental hospital, at least for a short period of time. Such patients, if such an abstraction is permissible, will tend to be men of the younger (under sixty) age-group. Most of them will be schizophrenics and when first seen at inception will have been ill for more than two years. One can see how all this might influence the decision for this kind of disposal. There will also be a certain amount of pressure coming from the family, who complain of the burden they have to carry, and this may be related particularly to the fact that dangerous behaviour appeared to be the clinical feature most commonly found in this group of patients.

It is most interesting that social class did not affect the different disposal between mental hospital and unit, except to a very slight degree in Class V. Classes I and II were as equally represented as Classes III and IV. This seems to be reassuring and shows that the service operates free of class pressures and gives proper opportunity for clinically appropriate decisions. It is also interesting that the older age-groups were by no means prone to go into mental hospital. They did require more in-patient treatment than the younger group, but this could be adequately provided in the units' own beds.

Patients admitted into mental hospital will also tend to be single men coming from the smaller household rather than the large one with five persons or more. Family groups, as one might expect, seem to have some protective effect, and the patients who have no one to lean on are the more exposed. One can see from a psychiatric point of view the patients who fall into this category are likely to be more difficult to manage in an extramural service.

Our findings are rather close to those reported by Zwerling and Wilder (1964), although they investigated a somewhat different extramural setting, with nevertheless similar problems. They studied a well-equipped day-hospital which aimed at avoiding in-patient admission, but had to resort to this on occasions. The day-hospital in their setting seemed in some ways comparable to a psychiatric unit in a general hospital, although the aim was even more ambitious: to work in the closest contact with the community from which their patients came. Zwerling and Wilder carried out a controlled study, allocating every other patient to a conventional type of management, where the decision to provide in-patient treatment was taken freely. In a sample of 189 psychiatric patients of all types, they found that 27% had to be transferred to in-patient care from the day-hospital after an attempt had been made to treat them there. The group that made up the 27% were very similar to our mental hospital admissions; they tended to be single, chronic male schizophrenics who showed dangerous behaviour and whose family seemed unable to cope with them at home.

We have mentioned the important roles played by the sense of 'subjective' burden and need for social care. These might well be expected, but we were to a certain extent surprised by the attitudes found amongst patients and their households towards the psychiatric units in general hospital and to mental hospital admission in particular. The expectation had been that one of the most favourable effects of these general hospital units would be the removal of stigma from psychiatric admission. The attitudes elicited show that this stigma had by no means been removed. Over one-half of the people who were asked still felt some reluctance over admission to the units, and the reluctance was slightly more widespread than towards admission to mental hospital. In fairness it could be said that this reluctance was no more perhaps than that which the public in general feel to admission to *any* hospital, but this question was not put and we know of no comparable study which would throw light on this point.

Yet when asked whether they felt in retrospect that the management of the patient's illness had seemed appropriate, the relatives on the whole appeared better satisfied if admission had actually been to the unit than to the mental hospital. This may, of course, be due to the fact that it tended to be the more difficult case who fell into the mental hospital group. The type of patient with an already chronic illness at the time of inception and therefore with hope fading considerably may have been the root of such dissatisfaction rather than the particular kind of management employed.

In spite of reluctance and prejudice against psychiatric admission in general, which if it had to be overruled gave rise to dissatisfaction amongst patients and relatives, there was in retrospect in many cases an appreciation of in-patient admission which had been experienced as helpful and appropriate to the patient's condition. In fact, when patients were kept out of hospital altogether in the four years under survey, the feeling that more could have been done or that the management might have been different was by no means absent. It may well have been that in these cases patients and relatives would have preferred in-patient treatment of any kind.

That such relief could be experienced, whatever the prejudice against admission might have been, was also reported by Grad and Sainsbury (1963) when they compared the Chichester extramural and Salisbury mental hospital services. In Salisbury, where patients were more readily admitted as in-patients than in the Chichester service, the sense of relief from burden was correspondingly higher.

The general conclusions that can be drawn are that an extramurally orientated type of psychiatric service will succeed all the better if in-patient treatment is not withheld at all costs, but used fairly liberally, particularly at the time of inception, when the illness is still a new experience for the household and the family members are still uncertain of what kind of help they are to expect from the service. Such a policy does not clash with the general goal of avoiding long-term hospitalization by all possible means; on the contrary, it will prepare the family much more thoroughly as to what they must expect, and make them perhaps more tolerant in their outlook as they become engaged in the task of looking after the incompletely recovered patient among them.

Whether the predictions that the mental hospital will disappear altogether will come true must depend on how well the psychiatric units can cope with this particular type of patient, who seems to have drifted into mental hospital care – namely, the young, disturbed chronic male schizophrenic, coming from the small household. The sheet-anchor, particularly of care for this type of patient, is still management rather than treatment, and the question will have to be faced of what further facilities the general hospital psychiatric units require to provide satisfactory long-term management for this type of patient and whether they can indeed provide it within their framework in the future.

CHAPTER V

Final Discussion and Conclusions

GENERAL

There can now be no doubt that these psychiatric units in general hospital provided a comprehensive psychiatric service to their catchment areas and largely satisfied the needs of their patients without recourse to prolonged stay in hospital, particularly in mental hospital. They seem, therefore, to be fulfilling the hopes that were initially vested in them. They did not cater for a selected group of patients, but looked after every type of psychiatric disorder, saw these patients, treated them, readmitted them, and apparently did this for the most part to the contentment of the patients and their relatives. 80% of the patients and 79% of the relatives in fact expressed themselves as satisfied with the service given by the units. In addition, all this had been achieved with very little recourse to the mental hospitals; indeed, over the four years only 0·7% of the patients became long-stay mental hospital patients.

The advantages of treating all or at least the vast majority of psychiatric patients in a general hospital are overpoweringly obvious, once it is established that this is possible in principle. The general hospital is within easy reach of the community from which patients come. This takes a good deal of the edge off admission: patients can be easily visited by relatives without too much time wasted on travelling. In the case of the two units we have surveyed, the respective mental hospitals presented a formidable journey for most relatives. Moreover, this cutting-off of patients from their own households is in itself a factor that may prolong in-patient stay and deepen isolation. Early discharge from a general hospital psychiatric bed is much less of a risk; relatives can come frequently and their opinions can be sought, and subsequent management discussed. Follow-up appointments at out-patient clinics can be arranged as a matter of course and the patient, his relatives, and the psychiatrist can derive reassurance from the fact that such follow-up contact is easier and the patient close at hand, so that readmission can be a relatively slight matter should the need arise. None of this occurs with the same facility if the hospital in question is miles away. Thus both admission and discharge seem smaller steps to take and may lead to more frequent in-patient admission, but also to a reduction in the length of stay. All this has been shown to be the case in these two units, where in-patient admission to the unit was resorted to in 66% of the patients, though 34% stayed less than one month and only 11% spent a total of more than three months in all over the four years, and of these only one patient stayed more than one year.

No doubt admission to mental hospital still carries a certain stigma, in spite of tremendous efforts that have been made to alter the character of these hospitals and educate the public to take a more objective view of them. In fact, the relatives did seem more satisfied if patients received all their treatment at the units than when a period of mental hospital treatment had been part of the four years' management. The stigma effect of mental hospital admission was undoubtedly on the wane, but it could not be said to have disappeared entirely. In fairness it must be remembered that some prejudice was also felt against admission to the psychiatric unit in the general hospital. It seems reasonable to assume that these general hospital units are in a better position to overcome this prejudice sooner, and we certainly found a move in their favour as the years went on.

The general hospitals themselves appeared to have welcomed the presence of the new psychiatric departments in a way not feasible twenty years ago. The units seem to have been accepted as part of the hospital service much as any other department and free use was made of mutual consultation. In fact, as many as 18% of all the referrals to the units came from consultants in other specialities.

The psychiatric patients themselves fitted easily into the general hospital framework. The dreaded vision that has sometimes haunted timid, conservative, and frequently ignorant physicians, surgeons, and administrators – the vision of noisy, unruly patients roaming about the hospital was dispelled – none of this came true. Instead, the psychiatric departments became fairly established as an integral part of the general hospital, and it would be fair to say that they would now be missed by the general hospital staff, who have come to rely on their participation in the day-to-day work. This co-operation was of mutual benefit at all levels of staff, as seems clear from the vivid description already given by the consultants-in-charge of the units. The presence of medical, surgical, obstetric, and gynaecological departments facilitated early investigation and treatment of physical illness in psychiatric patients, and ward consultations with psychiatrists in cases of attempted suicide, post-operative mental disorder, etc., frequently avoided transfer to special psychiatric beds in the hospital or in the mental hospital, by bringing psychiatric treatment to the general wards.

While most psychiatric patients only require in-patient care for very short periods, the units could accommodate longer-term patients too. For the very small number where this was necessary it could be done in the form of either in- or day-patient care. In this respect the units went beyond what was envisaged in the Hospital Plan of 1962, which the Minister of Health presented to Parliament. He then merely expected such units to deal with short-stay patients. In Section 27, p. 8, of that document, it is stated that '. . . it is now generally accepted that short-stay patients should be treated in units . . . attached to general hospitals'. Of course to what extent the longer-stay patients can be accommodated as the years go on, and should their numbers accumulate, will depend on the number of psychiatric beds per 1,000 population, which we discuss in the next paragraph. But as far as our present investigation goes, over the four years in question there seemed little sign of any large-scale silting up in this sense.

The important role which these general hospital psychiatric units are likely to play in the future psychiatric services is reflected in the Ministerial Hospital Plan, which provides for a general rundown of mental hospital beds. In the Manchester Hospital Board Region, of the 11,820 beds existing in 1960, there will be approximately 8,640 beds left in 1975, a decline of nearly 3,200 beds. Most of the beds are in the mental hospitals. In fact in 1960 only 1,578 psychiatric beds were in general hospitals, and in 1975 there will be slightly more – namely, 1,974. Thus, whereas mental hospital beds will be reduced in number by about one-third, the proportion of psychiatric beds in general hospitals will be increased. This means a reduction in the bed-population ratio of 2·7 beds per 1,000 population in 1960 to 1·9 in 1975. This latter figure, it will be noted, is slightly higher than the projected national average of 1·8 per 1,000 population. In 1960 the national average was 3·3 beds per 1,000 population, which was more than the figure for the Manchester Region. (These figures, of course, exclude the bed-numbers for mental subnormality.) Thus, whereas the Manchester Region was in terms of bed development slightly ahead of the country in 1960, its target for 1975 seems slightly less ambitious than for the rest of the country.

TABLE 103

Hospital plan: The Manchester region

	Number of Beds per 1,000 population	
	1960	1975
Acute	3·6	3·4
Geriatric	1·5	1·4
Maternity	0·47	0·56
Mental Illness	2·7	1·9

Table 103 shows the anticipated development in psychiatric beds in the Manchester Region in comparison with the anticipated development of other specialities.

A developed community care service has always been an integral part of the projected mental health services, and this was envisaged in conjunction with the general reduction of mental hospital beds and the proportionate rise of psychiatric beds in general hospitals. It was anticipated that the corollary to the curtailment of long-term hospital stay would have to be an expanded local authority service for psychiatric patients and their families. In discussing the future developments the report on the Hospital Plan for England and Wales says the following: 'This ratio [1·8 beds per 1,000 population] may well prove too high even if readmissions increase, for it takes no account of any contribution from the community mental health services or further advances in medical treatment... a ratio of 1·8 beds per 1,000 population has therefore been taken as the probable limit of requirements by 1975.'

Our investigation has shown that the local authority mental health services and other statutory social services were engaged in helping patients of these psychiatric units; but we also found that the help given was by no means exorbitant, and rarely reached anything but occasional help over the four years. On the whole, patients and families seemed satisfied with the amount of help received, and to a certain extent such help did appear directed towards those most in need. But at the same time there seems room for some further exploration to find out whether the services could not be more fully deployed, particularly in the matter of continuity of care after discharge from active treatment, and also to reach those who had difficulty in seeking help. Our inquiry gave the impression that such developments cannot be expected to come about spontaneously. Here is a largely unexplored field around these psychiatric units which calls for systematic research and perhaps a new kind of training for various personnel.

VULNERABLE PATIENT GROUPS

Once established, these psychiatric units by and large achieved what they had set out to do. It is, however, important to know whether the service did equally well for all groups of patients. It might generally be assumed that the extramural management would be more difficult for those patients who suffer from chronic, rather disturbing conditions, such as schizophrenia or organic psychosyndromes, than for patients whose illnesses tend to subside quickly. It might also be assumed that the service could do more for the younger patients, who tend to have more support from their families, may have less difficulty in returning to work, and are likely to suffer more from recoverable illnesses, than it could do for the elderly patients, who often live alone or in small households with another elderly or ageing person, who may not be able to give the necessary support. In the older age-group non-psychiatric illness often complicates the picture and adds to the difficulties of nursing and care in the home. It seems important therefore to locate such groups of patients and make a special effort to see whether the extramural type of psychiatric service provided adequately for them.

Schizophrenic Patients

The schizophrenic patient is in some ways the most interesting, as he presents the greatest challenge to this kind of management. It is not surprising that studies examining new schemes of psychiatric care tend to concentrate upon their effects on this particular diagnostic group, (Leyberg, 1965; Mandelbrote and Folkard, 1961*a*, *b*; Brown *et al.*, 1962; Wing *et al.*, 1964*b*; Shepherd, 1958; Waters and Northorer, 1965, etc.). The follow-up inquiry on our own sample showed that the schizophrenic patients were not too severe a challenge to the general hospital psychiatric unit. They tended to require in-patient treatment somewhat more frequently and for slightly longer periods than the psychiatric sample as a whole, but not markedly so. Nearly 15% never became in-patients at all during the four years and most of the admissions in any case took place at inception.

The figures for the total amount of time spent as in-patients in the unit, mental hospital, or both were striking. Less than 5% of the patients spent more than two years in all (not necessarily consecutively) and another 5% had spent from one to two years. In effect, therefore, 90% of the schizophrenic patients spent up to half of the follow-up time in the community. This pattern may be compared with that reported by Shepherd (1957), where practically all patients remained in mental hospital for the five-year follow-up period, once they have been admitted. The change in management for this diagnostic group of patients which our figures reflect is indeed one of the most striking changes that have appeared in the whole of psychiatric practice during the last decade.

But these psychiatric units in general hospitals seem to have achieved even more than other equally progressive services, based on mental hospital. This is suggested by the number of in-patients in the two different types of services at the end of the follow-up period. In one such service (Mandelbrote *et al.*, 1961*b*), 27·4% of the patients were still in mental hospital at the end of the follow-up period (four years), whereas in our own group of patients only 9·6%, i.e. one-third of the number, were found to be in-patients at the end of a similar period.

The fact that so large a proportion of schizophrenics can now be maintained outside hospital must not blind us to the high morbidity rate in terms of persistence of severe symptoms; this has not changed to the same extent over the years, if at all. Only about 25% of our group were free of symptoms for as long as three years, whereas nearly half (46·5%) were ill for two years or more. This state of affairs is far from satisfactory and reflects the inadequacy of the therapies at our disposal. On the other hand, we must remind ourselves that although this was a newly incepted group in the unit service, many of them had been ill before and were in fact already chronic patients. As we have shown earlier, these figures are no different from those for schizophrenic patients treated in other different types of psychiatric service.

Thus a picture finally emerges of patients, many of whom had remained ill through the major part of the follow-up period, yet who could be managed at home rather than in hospital. Many of them (well over one-third) worked for 75% of the period and only 30% remained completely unemployed throughout the four years. The figures for unemployment are still high if one thinks of the fate of the patient concerned, and one should not be complacent about them, but surely they are unexpectedly low for what one might expect in a chronically ill group such as this. The fact that a number of patients were in employment, however, must not be taken as completely reassuring, since in no less than 17% the current employment demanded less skill – in other words, the patients had declined in the social-class scale. Nevertheless, in general terms of work-adjustment our particular group of schizophrenic patients did do better than patients in the community-orientated services based on mental hospital, described by Mandelbrote and Folkard (1961) and Wing *et al.* (1964*b*).

It appears, therefore, that even progressive services, if based on mental hospital, are in some respects hampered as compared with those based on general hospital. The most likely explanation perhaps lies in the 'dampening-down' effect which mental hospital admission still tends to have on the spirits of patients, relatives, and employers, together with a number of advantages psychiatric units in general hospitals have over their mental hospital-based counterparts, as has been enumerated earlier.

Elderly and Aged Patients

The older age-group is sometimes expected to be difficult to manage in an extramural service, but our figures show this was not so. The patients in our sample over sixty years of age were indeed suffering, to a considerable extent – almost one-third – from organic psychosyndromes, while nearly half of them had serious physical illnesses in addition to the psychiatric disorder. Despite this, they did not remain as in-patients for any length of time, but were largely looked after in the community. Perhaps the difficulties arising from the gravity of their clinical condition tended to be offset by the high death-rate, which amounted to 39% of this group. But the death-rate, we hasten to add, could not be ascribed to the new type of extramural management, as we found it considerably lower than that among mental hospital patients in general.

19% of the over-sixty age-group never became in-patients at all, and of those who did the majority stayed less than three months in all during the four years. Only 6% had a total in-patient stay of more than one year. The mental hospital admitted just over 10% of those patients. Thus it seemed possible to keep most of these elderly patients in the community in the four years following their inception to the service, but free use was made of very short-term admissions, mainly to the general hospital psychiatric beds. Most of the admissions fell into the actual inception period. The express policy of the service appears to have succeeded not only better than might have been expected with this elderly group, but better than with other groups of patients. In fairness one must be careful of generalization here, as the proportion of geriatric patients seems to vary in different parts of the country; some of the success or otherwise may also be due to the extent non-psychiatric geriatric services are available in any given area, and to yet other factors as well.

There was, of course, a very high morbidity rate, although slightly less than with the under-sixty age-group. More than half of the older patients were ill for more than two years and only one-fifth had short-term illnesses, lasting less than six months. The remarkable thing is that, in spite of this adversity, the older group of patients did not experience long-term hospitalization in general and could be maintained for the most part in the community.

Thus even with the two most problematical groups of patients – the schizophrenics and the elderly – extramural care based on these psychiatric units in general hospital appears to have worked satisfactorily and achieved the desired results of the declared policy.

Contrasts between the Two Psychiatric Units

If the 'total hospital time' spent by our sample in-patients during the four years is compared in respect to the two psychiatric units separately, differences appear slight. But this apparent uniformity between the two unit populations reveals itself in parts as spurious on closer scrutiny. When the 'total hospital time' spent in mental hospital in the course of the four years is looked at separately, we find many more Blackpool patients were admitted than in Burnley – namely, 30% in Blackpool, but only 6% in the case of Burnley. As we have shown, the most important factor responsible for this difference was the shortage of general hospital psychiatric beds in Blackpool, so that the mental hospital beds were used for the overflow of patients and continued to be used for short-term admissions. They might therefore be seen in this sense as an extension of the unit. In Burnley the mental hospital admissions did not come about as an overflow phenomenon at all, but were the result of decisions made on grounds of a highly selective nature. In Blackpool, on the other hand, in the majority of such cases, the consultant appears to have had no other option.

We have seen that there were certain social and clinical differences which affected the patients in the two areas, but if these played any part at all in leading to this higher admission rate to mental hospital, it could only have been a very minor one. Our findings lead us to predict that if the psychiatric beds in the general hospital unit in Blackpool were to be increased to 0·4 beds per 1,000 population, instead of 0·13, as they were at the time of the survey, the mental hospital admission rate could be reduced to the level that prevailed in Burnley, or even lower if the psychiatrist-in-charge chose so to do.

In Blackpool, however, the average length of stay in mental hospital was somewhat longer than with the Burnley patients, or rather more patients fell into the longer-stay group. It is true that in Blackpool the numbers were small, but the difference between the practice of the two units remained a definite one. We think this is highly suggestive that mental hospital admission in itself has the effect of increasing the likely length of in-patient stay. Patients most prone to this effect will be patients with schizophrenia and organic psychosyndromes, single patients or those living on their own because widowed, separated, or divorced. This seems to underline once more that an extramural service based on psychiatric beds in general hospital is more likely to be highly effective than one based on a mental hospital, however progressive its outlook.

The accounts given earlier by the two consultants-in-charge of the units show that there were considerable socio-economic differences in the two catchment areas, and also make it clear that their own attitudes to the operation of such a service differed widely. It is most striking that, despite these contrasts, the stated policy of the extramural service succeeded to an equal extent in both areas; and apparently quite independently of these considerable differences.

Effects on the Patients

The policy of avoiding long-term hospitalization derives its main justification from the belief that it will protect the patient from institutionalization. But a situation where an only partially recovered person is encouraged to live in the community may bring other hazards. These cannot be dismissed off-hand and need investigation. On the other hand, keeping the patient as much as possible in the community may not only prevent institutionalization, but hold other positive benefits as well.

Here unfortunately we have no other exactly comparable study. We can only look at the effects on our patients in absolute terms. In some ways the picture which has emerged is not altogether discouraging; at the same time it indicates a degree of unsatisfactory circumstance which leaves no ground for complacency.

There was the encouraging finding that nearly half of the patients were mentally ill for less than six months, the majority of these less than one month (35%). On the other hand slightly more than one-third remained ill for at least two years and many for the entire period of the follow-up study. Furthermore, a good quarter of all the patients had non-psychiatric illness in addition, much of it chronic and lasting for two years or more. These are findings which show that many patients offer continuous problems; not much more perhaps could have been done for them, but until the matter is looked into more thoroughly, the possibility of more effective help cannot be dismissed. The death-rate, which was still higher than the general population, was certainly considerably lower than with a mental hospital population. There was no indication of any increased death-rate due to neglect or lack of hospital care. The same remarks apply to the suicide rate, which if anything showed a decrease in the areas since the general hospital psychiatric service had been introduced.

A good quarter of the patients of employable age were out of work for at least three years or more and approximately another 20% for more than half of the follow-up time – that is, nearly half of our sample were unemployed for the major part of the period. This rather high figure is perhaps not surprising if one keeps in mind the high morbidity rate and the stratification of the sample, but it seems that it might be improved.

Wing and his colleagues (1964*a*) have shown conclusively what scope there is in the way of work rehabilitation for very sick and deteriorated patients. Their recent study of discharged schizophrenics, involving careful predischarge selection and preparation and active co-operation of the rehabilitation services, of the Ministry of Labour, underlines the amount of planned effort that may be called for. Work rehabilitation of psychiatric patients does not follow automatically from avoidance of long-term institutional care, but requires a deliberate strategy. And if lasting results are to obtain, we have still, it seems, much yet to learn. About half our group of patients of working age were fully employed through the four years, although a number of them in less skilled jobs than before their illness. Women patients suffered particularly, not finding their way back into employment so readily as the men. Social Classes IV and V appeared to suffer the most, and clinical factors such as diagnosis and chronicity of illness before inception also played a part in the degree of readjustment to work. The consideration of factors such as these should prove useful when defining the most vulnerable groups of patients for prophylactic purposes.

Lastly, in view of the fact that so high a proportion of our patients (87%) were leading severely circumscribed lives at the time of inception, it was encouraging to find improvement taking place in the course of the four years, but the fact that a considerable amount of this restricted living still persisted at the time of follow-up (25% confined to home, 27% partly confined) would suggest that this is an aspect which calls for more careful scrutiny than our own broad inquiry could give it. One cannot otherwise say whether this degree of apparent 'social isolation' is to be taken as advantageous or harmful to the patient and his circle.

Effects on the Medical and Social Services

Medical Services

Having reassured ourselves that the predominantly extramural type of care had achieved what it set out to do and that the effects on the patients were not wholly unsatisfactory, although leaving room for improvement, the two reservations that sprang to mind were whether this type of service, which calls sparingly on the in-patient resources, did not do this either at the expense of the other psychiatric services or of the patients' families.

We were first of all interested to see how the psychiatric services other than the in-patient service were engaged. The out-patient sessions, which in the Blackpool unit have been described by the psychiatrist-in-charge as extremely harassing events with rarely less than ten to twenty patients at a time, did not seem to be dealing with the follow-up of patients to any large extent. 90% of the patients either never attended out-patients again or for fewer than ten times in the course of the four years; only 10% attended at a rate equivalent to once every two months. What is more, the figures were the same in both units. This could not be described as overtaxing the out-patient services. Furthermore, the figures show that it was not the patients who had the least in-patient treatment who used the out-patients more, but the other way round, i.e. those patients who required the most in-patient treatment also had more out-patient attendances. It would therefore convey a wrong picture to think of the situation as an undue transference of work from in-patient to out-patient services; the position was rather that when there was obviously a more seriously ill group of patients this required both forms of treatment; of the diagnostic groups, it was the schizophrenics who were over-represented here.

The day-hospital services were not very far developed at the time covered by our survey and they only played a relatively minor part in patient care; only 5% of the patients used them at all and one-half of these for short periods only. Analysis of cases showed, however, that without some such service the longer-term patients could not have been tolerated at home,and chronic in-patient stay would have been the only alternative.

Of the other general medical services, that of the general practitioner is the most important from our point of view. We recorded the patients' contacts with their general practitioner over the four years, irrespective of the reason, but we felt that most of them were connected with physical illness. About one-third of the patients were in regular contact, which meant at least once in two months. Here were found mostly the elderly patients, and those suffering from organic psychosyndromes, epilepsy and affective psychoses. The schizophrenics were conspicuously small in number. As far as comparison was possible, it seemed that the patients as a whole (all diagnoses) attended twice as often as the national average. Considering we were dealing with a group of patients selected by the fact that they had been referred to hospital specialists, one might well expect a higher usage of the general practitioner, but whether this figure would appear less if patients were kept longer in hospital is difficult to say. We do not know whether the demand on the general practitioner was larger for our sample than for non-psychiatric hospital referrals. It is interesting that the schizophrenic patients tended to be seen less often than the national average – namely, 4·5 times per annum, whereas the national figure is six times per annum, while for our cohort as a whole the figure was twelve times.

How often did the general practitioner have to approach the unit psychiatrist by re-referral of patients in the course of the four years? We found that re-referral occurred in just over one-quarter of the patients and in only 8% did this occur more than once. This does not seem to be a high figure, considering the amount of morbidity found. It would suggest that the general practitioners did not feel that treatment possibilities had been neglected or that there was still room for further treatment to be forthcoming. Similarly, the amount of domiciliary visiting consequent to that at inception was small and applied to only 4% of the patients. In the initial phase social class did not seem of relevance, but it had become a factor when repeated domiciliary visits were called for, visits appearing more frequently in Social Classes I and II.

Finally, the general hospitals of the area did not appear to be used in a covert way for the hospitalization of psychiatric patients, as seems to occur sometimes, especially with geriatric patients (Kidd, 1962*a*). One-fifth of our patients were admitted to general hospital over the four years, but only when physically ill and the great majority for short periods only.

It can therefore be said that neither the other psychiatric supporting services (out- and day-patient) nor the general medical services were landed with an undue amount of work over the four years, although comparative figures are lacking which would permit us to say precisely whether any increased usage had in fact occurred under this new type of management.

Social Services

The same picture prevailed with the social services. On the whole usage seemed very moderate. This was contrary to the general expectation that community care would involve more demands on supporting social care.

The local authority mental health services were undoubtedly the most engaged, but even here the help was mainly of an occasional nature: 28% of patients and families received such help; only 3% had frequent and substantial aid. As for the other statutory and voluntary services, their contribution can only be described as marginal. 85% of the patients received very occasional help or none at all. Of the remaining 15% periodic help was extended to 7% and relatively constant help to 8%. Of the households who received no social help (55%), only 11% said that they needed it; in their case 8% proved to have been reluctant to ask for help and 3% were ignorant how to go about it. It is interesting that the figures were similar in the two areas. Generally speaking, it seems to have been social rather than clinical factors which determined whether patients received this form of care.

There would seem to be room for amplification of these services; nevertheless, to the modest extent they were used, they were directed appropriately to the most needy, although 10% of the households who had no social service complained of severe 'subjective' burden. Co-ordination between the clinical and social services, particularly those for which the medical officer of health was responsible seemed well organized and a framework existed for continuity of care. This is indeed one of the fields where exact information is lacking and further research could throw valuable light on the question of how far and in what direction this social care should be extended, particularly as the Hospital Plan of the Ministry of Health refers to its important role in the future.

Effects on the Family

The most important apprehension regarding extramural care of psychiatric patients had surely been the fear that too much burden would devolve on the patient's family. Much valuable information has been gained through the pioneering work by Sainsbury *et al.* (1962) and by others, such as Brown *et al.* (1962), Wing *et al.* (1964*b*), Mandelbrote *et al.* (1961), etc. This work is still only in its beginnings and ways have yet to be discovered to make the various findings comparable.

Our own method of assessing burden has so far not been tested in other studies, but our results suggest that it possesses at least some validity. The most interesting finding was the discrepancy between what we have called 'objective' burden and the 'subjective' sense of burden experienced by the patient's household. Nearly half of the families (44·3%) did not carry any of the types of 'objective' burden recorded in this investigation, while 55·7% did. We do not know how this would compare with a group of psychiatric patients kept for long periods in mental hospital, nor do we know how it would compare with patients suffering from non-psychiatric illness. What we were able to do, however, was to examine a number of factors influencing the incidence of these two types of burden in our particular sample.

Of these factors the duration of the patient's illness seemed to be an important one. Not unexpectedly, the longer the patient remained ill, the more likely was it that some 'objective' burden would be created for his household. Different households seem to be variably affected. Patients living with their spouses seemed to occasion such burden in a greater number of cases than patients living with their parents. The relationship between 'objective' burden and the 'total hospital time' spent as in-patient proved to be a problematical one. It appeared that the longer the patient stayed in hospital, the more likely was it that 'objective' burden was present in his household. But we were not sure of the exact nature of this relationship. We thought, however, that the fact that the patient was causing such burden led to the longer hospital stay rather than the other way round, although the latter was not of course inconceivable. The negative aspect of this finding was perhaps of greater importance – namely, when patients did not go into hospital at all, or only for very short periods, this in itself did not increase the 'objective' burden on the household as defined here: that much must be considered as established.

In addition to assessing the 'objective' effects of the patient's illness on the household, we also inquired after the 'subjective' sense of burden which the families might have felt. Here we found that the two types of burden by no means coincided.

When 'objective' burden was very slight or non-existent, relatives had no sense of 'subjective' burden. Where there was a good deal of 'objective' burden of any kind, a very large number (about 75%) of the relatives expressed some sense of 'subjective' burden, but only one-fifth (19·6%) reported that this 'subjective' burden had been severe. The most interesting finding was that nearly a quarter of the households carrying a good deal of 'objective' burden made no complaints of any 'subjective' burden. We felt this particular discrepancy could be regarded as a somewhat crude yet useful measure of family tolerance towards the mentally ill in their midst. It is not an entirely unexpected finding and shows that the workability of an extramural type of psychiatric service depends very much on the attitudes prevailing among the public and not entirely on 'objective' criteria as to the amount of burden such management might create.

The sense of 'subjective' burden was experienced more severely among households where there were older patients and where patients were married. Patients who lived with their siblings seemed to be tolerated best, while those living with their grown-up children were tolerated least (again implicating the older age-group). More 'subjective' complaint appeared in the households of Social Classes I and II, though their 'objective' burden in fact proved to be the smaller. From the point of view of diagnosis, epileptics and those suffering from organic psychosyndromes were tolerated least by their households and patients with personality disorders tolerated best. The tolerance extended to schizophrenic patients, who, as we have shown, caused a good deal of 'objective' burden, was remarkably high. The duration of the illness was, of course, an increasing test on the family's goodwill, which tended to dwindle as time went on.

The crucial question of whether patients out of hospital gave rise to more 'subjective' burden in their households can be reassuringly answered in the negative. The findings were that the longer the patient had to stay in hospital, the greater the sense of 'subjective' burden in the family. This suggests that 'subjective' burden was one of the pressure factors which kept the patient in hospital. Again, it is the negative aspect of this finding which is of crucial importance – namely, when patients stayed out of hospital there was no increase in 'subjective' burden in the home. The extramural type of management was not the cause of 'subjective' burden as such, but the service was sufficiently sensitive to remove this burden from the household when it became too much to bear.

Attitudes of Patients and Relatives

Whereas the problem of family burden has begun to draw attention, the attitudes of patients and their households, whether they are satisfied or not and similar questions are still rather neglected. It has been perhaps too readily assumed that what seems to the doctor to be beneficial would appear in the same light to patients and relatives. Perhaps the subject has been neglected because of the dubious reliability of such attitude assessments in general. However, we thought this aspect of the inquiry deserved some attention.

We found that about 90% of the patients had in the first place the sympathetic support of their relatives in their illness. Among the 10% who did not enjoy this, those patients with personality disorders and epilepsy seemed to be rather numerous. Most schizophrenic patients enjoyed a measure of sympathy. This explains perhaps the relatively high degree of tolerance extended to them. It is not surprising that those patients who lacked sympathetic support from their households tended to stay in hospital longer. Again this demonstrates the sensitivity of the service to this type of family pressure. The above attitudes did not change substantially during the four years of follow-up.

We have seen that social agency care seemed on the whole directed to the families that needed it most, as indicated by complaints of 'subjective' burden. More interesting were the opinions which relatives held as to whether more might have been done for the patient during the four years. Of those who felt nothing more could have been done, 46·2% complained nevertheless of 'subjective' burden, most of them, it is true, of slight 'subjective' burden, but 8·2% of severe burden. This latter figure can be regarded as a measure of public expectation of service, or more accurately perhaps in this case of lack of expectation. From the point of view of doctors and administrators, such a situation represents a challenge. To make the service fully satisfactory, this particular group must be located and their situation studied in detail to see if there are not ways in which the severe 'subjective' burden can be eased.

Unwillingness to have the patient admitted as an in-patient to the psychiatric unit was expressed in 12% of the families; there was not much change in this proportion during the four years. Among the patients more than half had no positive attitude towards coming in, but many of them were too ill at the time to express a reliable opinion.

When patients were admitted as in-patients, in 56% the households had experienced great relief, and this was so in all cases where the family had reported severe 'subjective' burden, which is broadly consistent with the findings of Grad and Sainsbury (1963), who pointed up the relationship between hospital admissions and family relief.

Investigation into the overall question as to whether relatives and patients were satisfied with the service provided by the units showed that in each case some four-fifths expressed themselves as perfectly satisfied. Only 7% of the relatives and 1% of the patients had severe complaints to make. The relatives' complaints were the more numerous and some related directly to the extramural service; for instance, families felt a lack of support in their difficult task of looking after the patients at home. These were mainly the relatives of schizophrenic patients and patients with organic psychosyndromes. Although in this matter there is no room for complacency, the results as a whole must be regarded as gratifying, with 93% of the relatives expressing themselves as satisfied or venting only minor complaints, the majority of which were not related to the extramural service as such.

At the time of inception, objections to mental hospital admission were slightly more numerous among the relatives (22%) than the objections to unit admission (12%). But by the end of the four-year period, there was a striking increase in the objections to mental hospital (52%). It seemed that once the relatives had had the experience of the service provided by the unit, they were no longer so ready to accept mental hospital admission. As to the patients themselves, they were even more reluctant at inception and this negative attitude also increased over the four years.

Finally, when asked to give a retrospective opinion on whether anything more might have been done to help since their first contact with the psychiatric unit, only 9% of the relatives and 5% of the patients expressed the opinion that more might well have been done. The remainder were satisfied. It is not surprising to find that all those relatives who expressed some dissatisfaction had also complained of 'subjective' burden, which it is clear the medical and social services had not been competent enough to remove.

This probing of the attitudes among the relatives and patients produced on the whole encouraging findings, in that it showed that the new type of service had been acceptable to the vast majority of its clients. Both patients and relatives, particularly after having had some experience of the units' services, seemed on the whole to prefer the attention of the psychiatric unit to straightforward mental hospital admission.

Changed Role of the Mental Hospital

Although the attempt had been made by the units to avoid mental hospital admission wherever possible, it was clear that the mental hospital had remained to some extent a necessary part of the scene. We have seen that the figures for mental hospital admission for the two units together are a somewhat misleading measure of the extent to which unit policy had succeeded. The Burnley figures were quite different from those in Blackpool, and we have shown this to be largely due to the difference in the number of general hospital psychiatric beds available at the time of our survey. 0·4 beds per 1,000 population – which was the number available in the Burnley unit – seems to be the minimum prerequisite for successful application of the policy. The Burnley unit figures therefore will be more illustrative than those from Blackpool, where the unit did not possess this minimum number of beds.

Not more than 0·8% of the patients from the Burnley unit were in-patients in the mental hospital only; another 5% drifted in there over the four years after they had had in-patient treatment at the unit. Dr. Downham has said more about such cases in Chapter II, and hints at some of the reasons why these admissions had taken place. From his remarks, and also from the observations of Dr. Ferguson, it appears that mental hospitals might now begin to assume more specialist functions, admitting and treating specific kinds of patients, who can perhaps be looked after in special hospitals better than in general hospitals; this would apply to patients who present special security risks, or who require long-term custodial care because of the nature of their case – for example, drug addicts.

As regards the 'total hospital time' spent as in-patients in mental hospital, there was a higher incidence of longer-stay patients in the Blackpool area than in Burnley, if longer-stay is defined as more than one year. In fact, in Blackpool this occurred seven times more frequently than in Burnley. The difference may be due to many reasons, but we feel some of it was due to the fact that the mental hospital had to be used routinely more often than in Burnley (as explained above), and we suspect that the mental hospital was thus given more room to exercise its institutionalizing effect. These patients therefore tended to have a longer hospital stay than those who were mainly treated in the units. All the same, the patients who spent more than two years in all were a very small number indeed – only two patients, both in Blackpool and this amounted to no more than 0·7% of the total group.

The type of patient who tended to be admitted to mental hospital was the young, single man, usually suffering from schizophrenia and displaying dangerous behaviour, and who had been ill for more than two years already at the time of inception to the unit. It appeared, however, that it was not so much the actual 'objective' burden on the household that determined his admission, but the 'subjective' burden experienced by the family. This was particularly vividly illustrated in those patients who had never been in-patients in the units at all, but went straight to the mental hospital. In all these cases, the families complained of severe 'subjective' burden.

Generally speaking, the group of mental hospital patients presented social problems and attracted a significantly higher amount of social agency care. But there was a small group (10%) where social agency care had not been received, though need had been expressed. One cannot but suspect that more might well have been done for the families of these patients, and the smallness of the group should not detract from their importance, or lead one to ignore the severity of the problem they present.

On the whole both patients and relatives preferred treatment in the unit, but admission to both unit and mental hospital was appreciated as affording considerable relief. This finding was quite in line with that of Grad and Sainsbury (1963). There was, of course, a degree of dislike of mental hospital admission among the relatives and even more so amongst the patients. It was somewhat disappointing to find that much of this prejudice also existed in relation to the general hospital unit admissions. This might have been due to the novelty of these and more experience of the unit could dispel such prejudice. This hope seems to derive support from our finding that the rejecting attitudes towards unit admission diminished in the course of the four years, while the antagonism to mental hospital admission rose slightly in comparison.

In Chapter II Dr. Downham has described how he used the general hospital psychiatric unit to assist in the rehabilitation of patients who were already chronic long-stay patients in the mental hospital at the time our investigation began, thus illustrating the potentiality of these units to diminish the existing number of long-stay mental hospital patients, but we did not investigate the extent to which he had in fact succeeded, as this was outside our terms of reference. Apart from this, the activity of the new psychiatric units will certainly have a notable effect on the future of the mental hospitals, by taking over much of their work and preventing the new growth of long-stay populations. That this is already an operant process has been pointed out by Smith (1966). He writes:

It is perfectly true within the Manchester Region that the mental hospital population is running down. In the last eight years, for example, Lancaster Moor has gone down by nearly 1,000 patients and is now 190 off its 1975 target. Whittingham has gone down by about 750 and is now 350 off its 1975 target; Prestwich, which has a most extraordinarily difficult catchment area, vast in numbers and scattered in region, has gone down by over 500 patients in this time and is now just over 1,000 short of its 1975 target; Parkside has reduced by about 200 and is now 350 off its 1975 target. Thus there has been a reduction and in some cases resolution of the overcrowding, not by the units 'creaming the therapeutic potential',

but by their taking all cases and not using the mental hospital at all.
In the overall Hospital Plan [for England and Wales] there is envisaged a reduction in mental hospital beds; 20 hospitals are to disappear and others are to be reduced in size. The number of hospitals with 1,000 or more beds is to go down from 69 to 26. All this forecast was to come true by 1975.
Today, nine years off the target date, the picture shows a great deal of confusion. Some of the hospitals given the message of extinction have in fact slightly increased or retained their number of beds and are proceeding with an enhancement of their diagnostic and treatment facilities. Others, such as in the Manchester Region, are very much ahead of the run-down to their 1975 target.

From the above Smith draws the obvious conclusion that mental hospitals must justify their continuance by searching for new ways of fulfilling special needs. There are, for instance, groups of patients who would indeed benefit from care and study of their problems in special hospitals, e.g. epileptics, alcoholics, disturbed adolescents, certain types of personality disorder, drug-addicts, and many others. But all the time it is most important that a close organic link should continue and indeed increase in strength between the general and mental hospitals, whatever their future may be. Everything is to be gained by increasing the integration of the mental health service; nothing by its fragmentation.

Bibliography

A Hospital Plan for England and Wales (1963), Cmnd. 1,604, H.M.S.O., London.

Annual Report of the Board of Control, 1915–1920, H.M.S.O.

A Report of the Royal Commission on the Laws relating to Mental Illness and Mental Deficiency (1954–7), Cmnd. 169, London: H.M.S.O.

BLACKER, C. P. (1946), *Neurosis and the Mental Health Services*, Humphrey Milford, London: O.U.P.

BROOK, C. P. B. (1964), 'Psychiatric Units in General Hospitals', *Lancet*, II 684–6.

BROWN, G. W. (1959), 'Social Factors influencing Length of Hospital Stay of Schizophrenic Patients', *Brit. Med. J.*, II, 1300–2.

——, MOUCH, E. M., CARSTAIRS, G. M., and WING, J. K. (1962), 'Influence of Family Life on the Course of Schizophrenic Illness', *Brit. J. Prev. Soc. Med.*, XVI, 55–68.

CLARK, D. H. (1965), 'The Therapeutic Community Concept, Practice and Future', *Brit. J. Psychiat.*, CXI, 947–54.

FERGUSON, R. S., 'Side Effects of Community Care', *Lancet*, I, (1961), 931.

FREEMAN, H. L. (1960), 'Oldham and District Psychiatric Service', *Lancet*, I, 212–21.

GRAD, J., and SAINSBURY, P. (1963), 'Mental Illness and the Family', *Lancet*, I, 544–7.

HARE, E. H. (1955), 'Mental Illness and Social Class in Bristol', *Brit. J. Prev. Soc. Med.*, IX, 191–5.

HAMILTON, M. W., and HOENIG, J. (1966*a*), *The Extramural Service and the Mental Hospital*, 189–93.

—— (1966*b*), 'The Impact of an Extramural Service on Social Isolation', *Soc. Psychiat.*, I, 97–102.

—— (1966*c*), 'The Elderly Psychiatric Patient – Use of the Medical Services, *Med. Officer*, CXVI, 193–6.

HOENIG, J., and HAMILTON, M. W. (1965), 'Extramural Care of Psychiatric Patients', *Lancet*, I, 1322–5.

—— (1965), 'Social Agency Care of Schizophrenic Patients', *The Med. Officer*, CXIV, 303–6.

—— (1966*a*), 'A New Venture in Administrative Psychiatry, *Am. J. Psychiat.*, CXXIII, 270–9.

—— (1966*b*), 'The Schizophrenic Patient under New Management', *Comprehen. Psychiat.*, VII, 81–91.

—— (1966), 'The Schizophrenic Patient in the Community and His Effect on the Household', *Int. J. Soc. Psychiat.*, XII, 165–76.

—— (1966), 'The Burden on the Household in an Extramural Psychiatric Service', from *New Aspects of the Mental Health Services*, ed. H. Freeman, Pergamon Press.

—— (1966), 'Mortality in Psychiatric Patients', *Acta Psychiat. Scand.*, XLII, 349–61.

—— (1966), 'Elderly Psychiatric Patients and the Burden on the Household', *Psychiat. Neurol., Basel.*, CLII, 281–93.

—— (1966), 'Neue Entwicklungen im Gesundheitsdienst für Geisteskranke in Gross Britanien, *Fortschr. Neurol. Psychiat.*, XXXIV, 612–23.

—— (1967), 'Extramural Psychiatric Care and the Elderly', *Brit. J. Psychiat.*, CXIII.

HOENIG, J., and CROTTY, I. M. (1958), 'Some Aspects of the Work of a Regional Mental Hospital and of an Observation Ward', *Int. J. Soc. Psychiat.*, III, 260–77.

—— (1959), 'Psychiatric Patients in General Hospitals', *Lancet*, 122–3.

HOLLINGSHEAD, A. B., and REDLICH, F. C. (1958), *Social Class and Mental Illness*, New York.

INNES, G., and SHARP, G. A. (1962), 'A Study of Psychiatric Patients in North East Scotland', *J. Ment. Sci.*, CVIII, 447–56.

JONES, K. (1960), *Mental Health and Social Policy*, London: Routledge & Kegan Paul.

—— and SIDEBOTHAM, R. (1962), *Mental Hospitals at Work*, London: Routledge & Kegan Paul.

KAY, D. W. K., ROTH, M., and HALL, M. R. P. (1966), 'Special Problems of the Aged and the Organization of Hospital Services', *Brit. Med. J.*, II, 967–72.

KELLEY, F. E. (1964), 'Relatives' Attitudes and Outcome of Schizophrenia', *Arch. Gen. Psychiat.*, X, 389–94.

KESSEL, N., and HASSAL, C. (1965), 'Psychiatric Out-patients in Plymouth', *Brit. Med. J.*, II, 1491–5.

KESSEL, N. (1966), 'The Evaluation of the Plymouth Nuffield Clinic', the *Millbank Memorial Fund Quarterly*, Vol. XLIV, No. 1, 291–306.

KIDD, C. B. (1962*a*), 'Criteria for Admission of the Elderly to Geriatric and Psychiatric Units', *J. Ment. Sci.* CVIII, 68–74.

—— (1962*b*), 'Misplacement of Elderly in Hospital', *Brit. Med. J.*, II, 1491–5.

KREITMAN, N., 'Mental Disorder in Married Couples', *J. Ment, Sci.*, 108 (1962), 438.

LE GASSICKE, J., 'Psychotherapy', *Brit. Med. J.*, II (1966), 1,457.

LEIBERMAN, D. M., HOENIG, J., and AUERBACH, I. (1957), 'The Effect of Insulin Coma and E.C.T. on the 3-year Prognosis of Schizophrenia', *J. Neurol. Neurosnry. Psychiat.*, XX, 108–13.

LEYBERG, J. M. (1959), 'A District Psychiatric Service – the Bolton Pattern', *Lancet*, II, 282–4.

—— (1965), 'A Follow-up Study on Some Schizophrenic Patients', *Brit. J. Psychiat.*, CXL, 617–24.

LOGAN, R., and CUSHION, A. A. (1958), *Morbidity Studies from General Practice*, I, No. 14, H.M.S.O.

LOMAX, M. (1921), *The Experience of an Asylum doctor; with suggestions for Asylum and Lunacy Law reform*, London: G. Allen & Unwin.

MACLAY, W. S. (1958), 'Experiments in Mental Hospital Organisation', *Canad. Med. Ass. J.*, LXXVIII, 909–16.

MACMILLAN, D. (1956), 'An Integrated Mental Health Service', *Lancet*, II, 1,094.

MALZBERG, B. (1934), *Mortality amongst Patients with Mental Disease*, 234, Utica, N.Y.: State Hospital Press.

—— (1940), *Social and Biological Aspects of Mental Disease*, Utica, N.Y.: State Hospital Press.

MANDELBROTE, B. M., and FOLKARD, S. (1961*a*), 'Some Factors attached to Outcome and Social Adjustment in Schizophrenia', *Acta Psychiat. Scand.*, XXXVII, 223–35.

—— (1961*b*), 'Some Problems and Needs of Schizophrenics in Relation to a Developing Psychiatric Community Service', *Comps. Psychiat.*, 319–28.

MARSHALL, F. N., and PILE, G. R. (1953), 'Review of Mental Health Services, 1948–1953', files of the M.R.H.B.

'Memorandum on the Future Organisation of the Psychiatric Services' (1945), prepared jointly by the Royal College of Physicians, the British Medical Association, and the Royal Medico-Psychological Association, *Brit. Med. J. Supplement*, I, 111–16.

Ministry of Health (1944), *A National Health Service*, Cmnd. 6,502, H.M.S.O.

NORRIS, V. (1959), *Mental Illness in London*, London: Chapman & Hall Ltd.

Report by the Committee on Psychological Medicine of the Royal College of Physicians, London, January, 1963.

ROTH, M., and MORRISSEY, J. O. (1952), 'Problems in the Diagnosis and Classification of Mental Disorder in Old Age: with a Study of Case Material', *J. Ment. Sci.*, XCVIII, 66.

SAINSBURY, P., and GRAD, J. C. (1962), 'Evaluation of Treatment and Services', from *The Burden on the Community*, London: O.U.P.

—— (1963), 'Community Care and the Elderly Psychiatric Patient', *VIth Int. Congr. of Gerontology* (Person. Com.).

—— WALK, D., and GRAD, J. C. (1966), 'Evaluating the Graylingsell Community Psychiatric Service in Chichester; Suicide and Community Care', *The Millbank Mem. Fund Quart.*, XLIV, 243–78.

SHEPHERD, M. (1957), *A Study of the Major Psychoses in an English County*, London: Chapman & Hall.

—— (1958), 'The Social Outcome of Early Schizophrenia', *Psychiat. Neurol.* (Basel), CXXXVII, 224–9.

SILVERMAN, M. L. (1961), 'A Comprehensive Department of Psychological Medicine', *Brit. Med. J.*, II, 698–701.

—— (1965), 'A Comprehensive Department of Psychological Medicine; the Problem of the Day-patient Case-load: a 12 Months' Review', *Int. J. Soc. Psychiat.*, XI, 204–9.

SMITH, S. (1960), 'Review of the Psychiatric Units associated with General Hospitals in the Area of the Manchester Regional Hospital Board', report to the M.R.H.B.

—— (1966), 'The Manchester Plan for Psychiatric Services', *Brit. J. Psychiat.* (August Supplement), 5–6.

——, GIBB, G. M., and MARTIN, A. A. (1960), 'Metamorphosis of a Mental Hospital', *Lancet*, II, 592–3.

—— (1963), 'Using Mental Hospitals for Other Purposes', *Lancet*, II, 398–400.

'The Royal Commission on Lunacy and Mental Disorder (1926)', Cmnd. 2,700, London: H.M.S.O.

WATERS, M. A., and NORTHORER, J. (1965), 'Rehabilitated Long-stay Schizophrenics in the Community', *Brit. J. Psychiat.*, CXI, 258–67.

WING, J. K., BENNETT, D. H., and DENHAM, J. (1964), 'The Industrial Rehabilitation of Long-stay Schizophrenic Patients', *Med. R.C. Memorand.*, 42, London: H.M.S.O.

——, MONCK, E., BROWN, G. W., and CARSTAIRS, G. M. (1964), 'Morbidity in the Community of Schizophrenic Patients discharged from London Mental Hospitals in 1959', *Brit. J. Psychiat.*, CIX, 10–21.

ZWERLING, J., and WILDER, J. E. (1964), 'Evaluation of the Applicability of the Day-hospital in Treatment of Acutely Disturbed Patients', *Israel. Au. Psychiat.*, II, 162–85.

Index of Authors

Index

For Product Safety Concerns and Information please contact our EU representative GPSR@taylorandfrancis.com
Taylor & Francis Verlag GmbH, Kaufingerstraße 24, 80331 München, Germany

www.ingramcontent.com/pod-product-compliance
Ingram Content Group UK Ltd.
Pitfield, Milton Keynes, MK11 3LW, UK
UKHW022110190926
475702UK00013B/1371
9780415864169